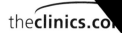

theclinics.com

FOOT AND ANKLE CLINICS

Complex Salvage of Ankle and Hindfoot Deformity

GUEST EDITORS
John G. Anderson, MD
Donald R. Bohay, MD

CONSULTING EDITOR
Mark S. Myerson, MD

March 2007 • Volume 12 • Number 1

SAUNDERS

An Imprint of Elsevier, Inc.
PHILADELPHIA   LONDON   TORONTO   MONTREAL   SYDNEY   TOKYO

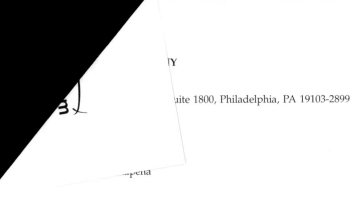

Y

uite 1800, Philadelphia, PA 19103-2899

...peña

Volume 12, Number 1
ISSN 1083-7515
ISBN 1-4160-4312-8
978-1-4160-4312-6

Foot and Ankle Clinics (ISSN 1083-7515) is published quarterly by Elsevier, Inc., 360 Park Avenue South, New York, NY 10010-1710. Months of issue are March, June, September, and December. Business and Editorial Offices: 1600 John F. Kennedy Blvd., Suite 1800, Philadelphia, PA 19103-2899. Customer Service Office: 6277 Sea Harbor Drive, Orlando, FL 32887-4800. Periodicals postage paid at New York, NY, and additional mailing offices. Subscription prices are $314.00 per year Institutional, $270.00 per year Institutional USA, $314.00 per year Institutional Canada, $253.00 per year Personal, $187.00 per year Personal USA, $209.00 per year Personal Canada, $121.00 per year Personal student, $94.00 per year Personal student USA, $121.00 per year Personal student Canada. To receive student/resident rate, orders must be accompanied by name of affiliated institution, date of term, and the *signature* of program/residency coordinator on institution letterhead. Orders will be billed at individual rate until proof of status is received. Foreign air speed delivery is included in all *Clinics* subscription prices. All prices are subject to change without notice. POSTMASTER: Send address changes to *Foot and Ankle Clinics*, Elsevier Periodicals Customer Service, 6277 Sea Harbor Drive, Orlando, FL 32887-4800. **Customer Service: 1-800-654-2452 (US). From outside of the US, call 1-407-345-1000.**

Printed in the United States of America.

CONSULTING EDITOR

MARK S. MYERSON, MD, President, American Orthopaedic Foot and Ankle Society; Director, Institute for Foot and Ankle Reconstruction, Mercy Medical Center, Baltimore, Maryland

GUEST EDITORS

JOHN G. ANDERSON, MD, Associate Professor, Department of Orthopaedic Surgery, Michigan State University, College of Human Medicine, Orthopaedic Associates of Grand Rapids, Grand Rapids, Michigan

DONALD R. BOHAY, MD, FACS, Associate Professor, Department of Orthopaedic Surgery, Michigan State University, College of Human Medicine; Orthopaedic Associates of Grand Rapids, Grand Rapids, Michigan

CONTRIBUTORS

LUCILLE B. ANDERSEN, MD, Assistant Professor, Penn State Milton S. Hershey Medical Center, Orthopaedics and Rehabilitation, Penn State College of Medicine, Hershey, Pennsylvania

VIKRANT AZAD, MD, Research Associate, Department of Orthopaedic Surgery, New Jersey Medical School—University of Medicine and Dentistry New Jersey, Newark, New Jersey

JUDITH F. BAUMHAUER, MD, Professor and Chief, Division of Foot and Ankle Surgery, Department of Orthopaedics, University of Rochester Medical Center, Rochester, New York

CHRISTOPHER BIBBO, DO, Director, Foot and Ankle Service, Department of Orthopaedics, Marshfield Clinic; Clinical Instructor, Department of Orthopaedics and Rehabilitation, University of Wisconsin School of Medicine, Marshfield, Wisconsin

ERIK CALVERT, MD, FRCSC, Foot and Ankle Fellow, Division of Lower Extremity Reconstruction and Oncology, Department of Orthopaedics, University of British Columbia, Vancouver, British Columbia, Canada

BENEDICT F. DIGIOVANNI, MD, Associate Professor, Division of Foot and Ankle Surgery, Department of Orthopaedics, University of Rochester Medical Center, Rochester, New York

A. SAMUEL FLEMISTER, MD, Associate Professor, Division of Foot and Ankle Surgery, Department of Orthopaedics, University of Rochester Medical Center, Rochester, New York

PAUL T. FORTIN, MD, Attending Surgeon, Department of Orthopaedic Surgery, William Beaumont Hospital, Royal Oak, Michigan

TOMIKO FUKUDA, MD, Resident, Department of Orthopedic Surgery, Northwestern University Memorial Hospital, Northwestern University, Chicago, Illinois

VIC GIBSON, DO, Orthopedic Resident, Department of Orthopedic Surgery, Botsford General Hospital, Farmington Hills, Michigan

TODD A. IRWIN, MD, Resident, Department of Orthopaedic Surgery, William Beaumont Hospital, Royal Oak, Michigan

PAUL J. JULIANO, MD, Professor, Penn State Milton S. Hershey Medical Center, Orthopaedics and Rehabilitation, Penn State College of Medicine, Hershey, Pennsylvania

JOHN KOERNER, MS, Medical Student, New Jersey Medical School—University of Medicine and Dentistry New Jersey, Newark, New Jersey

JOSEPH X. KOU, MD, Resident, Department of Orthopaedic Surgery, William Beaumont Hospital, Royal Oak, Michigan

SUSAN MOSIER LACLAIR, MD, Clinical Assistant Professor, Department of Orthopaedic Surgery, Michigan State University; Family Orthopedic Associates, Flint, Michigan

SHELDON S. LIN, MD, Associate Professor, Department of Orthopaedic Surgery, Foot and Ankle Division, New Jersey Medical School—University of Medicine and Dentistry New Jersey, Newark, New Jersey

FRANK A. LIPORACE, MD, Assistant Professor, Department of Orthopaedic Surgery, Trauma Division, New Jersey Medical School—University of Medicine and Dentistry New Jersey, Newark, New Jersey

KENNETH R. MORSE, MD, Resident, Department of Orthopaedics, University of Rochester Medical Center, Rochester, New York

SCOTT NEMEC, DO, Orthopedic Resident, Department of Medical Education, Ingham Regional Medical Center, Michigan State University; College of Osteopathic Medicine, Lansing, Michigan

MURRAY PENNER, BSc (MEng), MD, FRCSC, Surgeon, Foot and Ankle Program, Providence Health Care, Clinical Associate Professor, Division of Lower Extremity Reconstruction and Oncology, Department of Orthopaedics, University of British Columbia, Vancouver, British Columbia, Canada

DAVID PRIESKORN, DO, Tri County Orthopedics, Farmington Hills, Michigan

AMY JO PTASZEK, MD, Clinical Instructor, Northwestern University Medical School, Illinois Bone and Joint Institute, Ltd., Glenview, Illinois

VERRABDHADRA REDDY, MD, Resident, Department of Orthopedic Surgery, Northwestern University Memorial Hospital, Northwestern University, Chicago, Illinois

MICHAEL P. STAUFF, MD, Penn State Milton S. Hershey Medical Center, Orthopaedics and Rehabilitation, Penn State College of Medicine, Hershey, Pennsylvania

MICHAEL P. SWORDS, DO, Assistant Clinical Professor, Michigan State University College of Osteopathic Medicine, Mid Michigan Orthopaedic Institute, East Lansing, Michigan

ANTHONY D. WATSON, MD, Greater Pittsburgh Orthopaedic Associates, Pittsburgh, Pennsylvania

TROY S. WATSON, MD, Director, Foot and Ankle Institute, Desert Orthopaedic Center, Las Vegas, Nevada

ALASTAIR YOUNGER, MB, ChB, MSc, ChM, FRCSC, Director, Foot and Ankle Program Providence Health Care, Clinical Associate Professor, Division of Lower Extremity Reconstruction and Oncology, Department of Orthopaedics, University of British Columbia, Vancouver, British Columbia, Canada

CONTENTS

Ankle arthritis is a commonly seen problem. Numerous treatment options exist. The role of osteotomies of the tibia, fibula, midfoot, and hindfoot and their applications in the treatment of ankle arthritis are discussed.

The valgus ankle is a complex deformity with many possible origins. The most common cause, however, is degenerative in the form of untreated chronic posterior tibial tendon dysfunction. Regardless of the cause, the principles of treatment remain the same: One must attempt to achieve a painless, plantigrade foot while preserving maximal flexibility. Various options are available for treatment, including osteotomies, fusions, and arthroplasty. Each has its own advantages and disadvantages. The valgus ankle can lead to severe deformity, debility, and pain, stressing the importance of optimal management of this condition. This article reviews the entity of the valgus ankle, discusses its clinical recognition, and reviews forms of treatment.

procedures with consistent results. Unfortunately, many potential complications have been cited throughout the literature. Although the most important aspect in any fusion surgery is meticulous technique, advances in technology, including platelet-rich plasma, bone stimulators, and bone morphogenetic proteins, seem to be useful additions in the quest to achieve solid fusions with decreased complications.

Open treatment of calcaneal fractures has increased in popularity overthe past 10 to 15 years among orthopaedic surgeons but remains controversial secondary to the associated complications. In the literature, the most common soft tissue complications following calcaneal fractures include wound necrosis, compartment syndromes of the foot leading to late deformity, chronic pain from neurovascular injury, and various tendon problems. The initial evaluation of the patient who has a calcaneal fracture prior to operative treatment may reduce the incidence of postoperative complications by identifying and rectifying risk factors. In some cases, nonoperative treatment may be indicated to avoid disastrous postoperative wound issues and deep infection.

Though the debate continues between operative interventions versus conservative therapy, there is significant evidence that the deformity that results from calcaneus malunions causes significant disability for the patient. Knowledge of the fracture patterns in the original calcaneal fracture aids in both understanding the deformity of the malunion and the necessary steps for correction of the deformity.

Talar injuries present a unique set of challenges because of the precarious blood supply and its special function. Restoring anatomy is extremely important but does not necessarily exclude poor outcome because avascular necrosis, malunion, and posttraumatic arthritis are common sequelae. The reconstructive options for avascular necrosis and posttraumatic arthritis are numerous. Anatomic reduction of varus malunions is an effective treatment in the face of normal adjacent joints.

FORTHCOMING ISSUES

RECENT ISSUES

THE CLINICS ARE NOW AVAILABLE ONLINE!

http://www.theclinics.com

ELSEVIER
SAUNDERS

Foot Ankle Clin N Am
12 (2007) xiii–xiv

FOOT AND
ANKLE CLINICS

Foreword

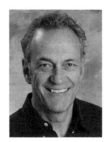

Mark S. Myerson, MD
Consulting Editor

Over the past decade the approach to treatment of ankle injury and arthritis has evolved. Yet despite the significant expansion of these treatment alternatives, most of these procedures are nonetheless performed as a means of salvaging arthritis. Ankle arthrodesis, joint replacement, or osteoarticular allografts are not joint-preserving methods of treatment, and the biomechanics of the hindfoot and ankle are never restored. It is reassuring however to note that treatments aimed at joint preservation are gaining popularity. For example, the goal of supramalleolar osteotomy and ankle distraction arthroplasty is to maintain, preserve, and hopefully improve joint function. If one examines further the alternative methods of articular preservation, cartilage stimulation has not yet received sufficient attention in the foot and ankle. We are slowly gaining an understanding into these alternative biologic treatments of articular cartilage deficits with oral medication, electrical stimulation, and even shock wave therapy. These modalities may be primary or adjunctive to longer term surgical planning, but should become part of our armamentarium for the management of arthritis of the foot and ankle. Adequate correction of deformity is essential when one hopes to restore articular function; the articles on the malunited calcaneus, talus, and distal tibia fractures give an excellent approach to this problem. Although salvage of severe ankle arthritis may necessitate either joint

1083-7515/07/$ - see front matter © 2007 Elsevier Inc. All rights reserved.
doi:10.1016/j.fcl.2007.01.001
foot.theclinics.com

replacement or arthrodesis, these should be part of and not the only treatment options selected by the orthopedic surgeon.

Mark S. Myerson, MD
Institute for Foot and Ankle Reconstruction
Mercy Medical Center
301 St. Paul Place, Baltimore
MD 21202, USA

E-mail address: mark4feet@aol.com

ELSEVIER
SAUNDERS

Foot Ankle Clin N Am
12 (2007) xv–xvi

FOOT AND
ANKLE CLINICS

Preface

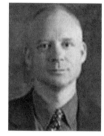 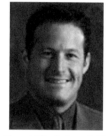

John G. Anderson, MD   Donald R. Bohay, MD
Guest Editors

The modern day foot and ankle surgeon is facing a growing number of complex degenerative and posttraumatic conditions, which have by necessity, spurred the growth in our subspecialty in both number of procedures performed and number of providers. Concomitantly, society has placed greater demands on our subspecialty to deliver superior quality of care and ensure restoration of a high level of function. By nature of the relative infrequency of which certain complex conditions are seen in any individual's office, our ability to share meaningful information and experiences becomes critical in the advancement of our science and in the promotion of our members.

It is not unusual for the foot and ankle subspecialist to be one of the busiest physicians in his/her community. This is only partly explained by the growing population and increasing incidence of foot and ankle disorders. Another key factor is our ability to correct and improve upon conditions that were previously unrecognized or felt to be uncorrectable. Clearly our focus on advancing technology and improving outcomes has led to tremendous strides in treatment of the foot and ankle in the last 10 to 15 years. The growth in publications with emphasis on the foot and ankle is testimony to our progress.

This edition of *Foot and Ankle Clinics* was put together with the intent of bringing to the forefront some of the advances we have witnessed with regard to salvage of complex ankle and hind foot disorders. We believe we have put together a panel of authors who have demonstrated excellence throughout their young careers and who have a desire to move our

doi:10.1016/j.fcl.2006.12.005

subspecialty into the next era. We have witnessed the progression of our specialty from one whereby success is determined not just by the presence of union and absence of infection, but also by proper maintenance of alignment, preservation of essential motion, restoration of stability, providing of pain relief, and improvement of function, all while preserving footwear options. Although all these goals are the ideal, and clearly they cannot always be achieved, we have made great strides in our collective performance over the course of our professional careers. For example, the use of osteotomies and tendon rebalancing procedures to restore alignment while preserving motion, the use of rigid fixation to achieve union, and the recent use of bioadjuvants are all areas whereby tremendous progress has occurred.

This issue addresses some of the challenging problems we all face and struggle with, and we hope you find it helpful in guiding you through your clinical practice. We thank all the fine people at Elsevier as well as Dr. Mark Myerson for their assistance with putting this edition together. We would also like to especially thank all of the authors for their valuable time and expertise. As we find our subspecialty growing in numbers and technical expertise, our hope is that the future holds even greater advances that we may at present think unimaginable.

John G. Anderson, MD
and
Donald R. Bohay, MD
Department of Orthopaedic Surgery
Michigan State University
College of Human Medicine
Orthopaedic Associates of Grand Rapids
1111 Leffingwell NE, Suite 100
Grand Rapids, MI 49525, USA

E-mail addresses: jganderson@oagr.com;
drbohay@oagr.com

ELSEVIER
SAUNDERS

Foot Ankle Clin N Am
12 (2007) 1–13

FOOT AND
ANKLE CLINICS

Osteotomy for Salvage
of the Arthritic Ankle

Michael P. Swords, DO[a],*, Scott Nemec, DO[b]

[a]Mid Michigan Orthopaedic Institute, Michigan State University College of Osteopathic
Medicine, 830 West Lake Lansing, Suite 190, East Lansing MI 48823, USA
[b]Department of Medical Education, Ingham Regional Medical Center, Michigan State
University College of Osteopathic Medicine, 401 West Greenlawn Avenue,
Lansing MI 48901, USA

Supramalleolar osteotomy

Osteotomies for correction of foot and ankle malalignment are well described in the literature for treatment of congenital and acquired pediatric disorders [1–6]. Less well documented is the use of osteotomies for the treatment of ankle arthritis. Osteotomies in the tibia or foot, alone or in combination, can be used for ankle arthritis. Long-term studies following tibial shaft fractures with malunion vary in the role of malunion on the function of the ankle and arthritis. Merchant and Dietz [7] followed 37 tibia shaft fractures to a mean of 29 years postinjury. Some 78% of patients had good results both clinically and radiographically in the ipsilateral ankle. Fourteen patients had a malunion of greater than 10°. Puno and colleagues [8] evaluated 27 patients at an average of 8 years after a tibia shaft fracture and found patients who had greater malorientation of the ankle joint had worse outcomes. Milner and colleagues [9] followed 164 tibia shaft fractures at a mean of 36 years after injury. Various malunions were present in the study population. Patients displayed excessive pain with passive motion and objective stiffness in both the ankle and subtalar joints. At the time of follow-up no patient had undergone a surgical procedure for ankle arthritis.

Simulated malunions seem to alter contact pressure within adjacent joints. These changes seem to increase as the malunion is placed in closer proximity to the joint [10]. Changes in biomechanics of the tibiotalar joint with respect to contact pressures result when angular deformities of the distal tibia are present. Tarr and associates [11] demonstrated up to 42%

---

* Corresponding author.
E-mail address: foot.trauma@gmail.com (M.P. Swords).

doi:10.1016/j.fcl.2006.11.002
foot.theclinics.com

decrease in contact pressures with apex anterior angulation of 15°. The study also indicated that 10° to 15° angular deformity in any plane tended to elongate the contact area and shift the area laterally. Malalignment of 15° or less for proximal and midshaft tibial fractures showed no alteration in contact patterns. Varus deformity is less tolerated than valgus deformity as a result of greater compensatory inversion versus eversion, 20° to 5° respectively, at the subtalar joint [11]. Simulated subtalar stiffness increases the mechanical alterations of the ankle after malunion [10]. As a result, a lower threshold for performing supramalleolar osteotomy for varus deformities is recommended over valgus deformity. Left untreated the abnormal wear may lead to severe arthritis, requiring either arthroplasty or arthrodesis for definitive management. Osteotomies provide an opportunity to correct malalignment and address secondary arthritic issues. Changing wear patterns by realignment procedures is beneficial to joint preservation and function by unloading damaged cartilage and loading healthy cartilage [12,13]. Pain resulting from a localized area of arthritic change may be improved by shifting contact characteristics more evenly across a broader joint surface area.

The type of osteotomy to be performed is determined by the deformity, the condition of surrounding soft tissues, current leg length issues, and status of the articular surface. Closing wedge osteotomies are the most commonly performed osteotomy. This technique is typically applied directly to the center of rotation. Because of the compression of the resultant osteotomy surfaces, bone graft is usually not required. Potential problems with closing wedge osteotomies include soft tissue complications attributable to a larger exposure, especially in the posttraumatic population. Additionally, removal of the bone segment can alter desired effects on leg length if not carefully planned. This outcome is usually offset by the improvement in leg length achieved with the correction of deformity. An opening wedge osteotomy allows for maintaining or increasing length and can typically be performed with smaller dissection than closing wedge osteotomies. Leg length has been shown to be better preserved with the use of an opening wedge osteotomy [14]. Of concern is the creation of a large triangular defect that typically requires some form of bone graft and can potentially increase the risk for nonunion. Stamatis and colleagues [13] found that there were lower rates of nonunion with closing wedge osteotomies, whereas Takakura and colleagues [15] found less chance of nonunion in opening wedge osteotomies. Both forms of osteotomy have the potential to alter the functional length of tendons required for optimum motor function. If correction requires addressing both angulation and rotational deformity this can still be addressed using a single-cut osteotomy. This can be calculated using mathematical formulas [16]. A cut through the bone in the horizontal plane corrects rotational issues. If a cut is made in the long axis of the tibia in the coronal plane the varus/valgus can be corrected. The mathematical formula allows for the preoperative evaluation and surgical planning to accurately predict the single-cut osteotomy required to correct both aspects of the deformity and has been used successfully to treat a small clinical series [16].

Osteotomies require preoperative planning. The type and location of the osteotomy should be based on long leg radiographs. Any malalignment of the hindfoot or equinus should be addressed at the same setting. It is imperative to assess subtalar range of motion to determine if the joint will tolerate the new alignment. Arthroscopy or arthrotomy may be performed at the beginning of the procedure to be sure there is enough viable articular cartilage for the osteotomy to be successful [12]. The plane of the deformity is determined in the operative setting by using fluoroscopy to find the view of the tibia with no visible deformity. The plane of the deformity is orthogonal to this plane. K wires may be inserted to act as reference guides when cuts are made. The first wire is inserted horizontally across the shaft perpendicular to the long axis. A second wire can be inserted parallel to the ankle mortise. The deformity is then corrected by using either a closing or opening osteotomy, depending on the deformity. Care is taken to maintain a hinge at the far cortex to avoid translation. Opening wedge osteotomy requires a single saw cut parallel to the articular surface. Closing wedge osteotomy requires the saw cuts that are in the same plane if correction lies in a single plane. If a second plane of deformity is being addressed the cuts must be oriented to resect additional bone anteriorly or posteriorly. Opening wedge osteotomies in the distal tibia are usually approached medially, whereas closing wedge osteotomies can be performed from either lateral or medial with osteotomy of the fibula through the same incision or through a second lateral incision.

When looking at supramalleolar osteotomies for the correction of angular deformity, postosteotomy stabilization must be strong enough to obtain and maintain the correction over time. In children stabilization can be acquired with the use of Kirschner wires or staples in conjunction with casting, or with casting alone. In treating the adult population this does not provide sufficient fixation. External fixation, plates and screws, and intramedullary fixation are all possible routes of stabilization, with each yielding beneficial aspects. Small wire fixators are beneficial in cases in which acute correction of the deformity is not possible or infection prevents the use of internal fixation. Numerous reports detail the use of Ilizarov frames for the fixation of supramalleolar osteotomies and late correction of deformity, so further discussion of this method is not included here.

Modern plate design has made plating in this anatomic region easier. Several manufacturers market precontoured plates for the distal tibia. Plates matching the anatomy of the anterolateral and medial aspects of the tibia are readily available. Precontoured plates are generally lower profile and allow for more screws to be inserted in close proximity to the distal tibia articular surface than standard plates. Plates with locking screw options are also available and may be of benefit in cases with poor bone density or posttraumatic bone loss. Patients who have plate and screw fixation are generally non–weight-bearing for 8 to 12 weeks.

Intramedullary nail fixation is also an option for osteotomies in the distal third of the tibia (Fig. 1). Modern nail design allows for more distal insertion of locking bolts and bolts in multiple planes. With respect to intramedullary nailing, osteotomy sites are generally more proximal than those osteotomies addressed with plates and screws. The benefits of intramedullary nailing are derived from the ability of the device to load share, which allows significantly earlier weight-bearing than with plate and screw constructs. Contraindications for the use of intramedullary nails include large deformities that would not allow a straight device to pass down the canal once corrected, very distal or intra-articular involvement that would limit the ability to adequately secure the distal segment, the need for translation of a bone segment, and a desire by the surgeon or the patient to avoid

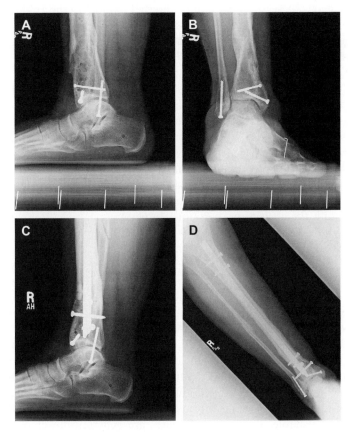

Fig. 1. This patient is a 34-year-old woman who has posttraumatic arthritis because of a malunited pilon fracture sustained in a motor vehicle accident. (A, B) Preoperative images show an extension malunion with significant anterior impingement. The mortise shows moderate arthritis. (C, D) A closing wedge osteotomy was performed to correct the tibial malalignment. An oblique osteotomy was made through the fibula. The patient was allowed to bear weight at 2 weeks. Postoperatively the patient had improvement in her arthritic pain.

potential complications at the knee. When using nail fixation for osteotomies, provisional fixation can be achieved by a unicortical plate at the site of osteotomy or by using a simple temporary external fixator. The external fixator can be a simple two-pin construct with one pin inserted in the proximal tibia posterior to the nail entry site. The second pin is placed parallel to the distal tibia articular surface and parallel to the deformity. After osteotomy the pins are rotated until parallel and then the frame is locked, securing the osteotomy site while the intramedullary implant is placed. Alternatively a universal femoral distractor may be used. Compression of the osteotomy site can be obtained through the distractor or by using the compression distractor device standard in the large external fixator set. Care must be taken not to introduce additional deformity by errant pin placement.

Results

Few series on supramalleolar osteotomies have been reported, but results have generally been favorable. Takakura and colleagues [12] reported on 18 patients treated with supramalleolar osteotomy for intermediate-severity arthritis of the ankle. All were performed to treat varus malalignment. To compensate for arthritic changes the osteotomy was performed to slightly overcorrect so as to shift more weight-bearing onto the better articular cartilage in the lateral portion of the ankle. Arthroscopy was performed at the beginning of the procedure to confirm arthritic findings medially and better cartilage in the lateral ankle. Follow-up averaged 6 years 11 months (range 2.7–12.10 years). Results were excellent in 6, good in 9, and fair in 3, with no poor results. Arthroscopic examination was performed in 10 patients with development of fibrocartilage medially in 7. The authors concluded that osteotomy with slight overcorrection was effective in treating intermediate ankle arthritis.

Takakura and colleagues [17] also published a series of nine patients treated with opening wedge osteotomies for posttraumatic varus deformity of the ankle. Four patients had an excellent result, two had a good result, and three had a fair result. A decrease in range of motion was seen in six patients.

Stamatis and colleagues [13] reported on 12 patients treated with supramalleolar osteotomy for distal tibial malalignment of at least 10° and pain. Eight patients had arthritis preoperatively. Follow-up averaged 33.6 months. The average AOFAS score improved from 53.8 to 87. In this short follow-up period they did not see any progression of radiographic findings of arthritis.

Fibular osteotomies

Isolated fractures of the lateral malleolus or those occurring as part of a more complex injury pattern are commonly seen injuries. The lateral malleolus has been described as the key to the ankle joint [18,19]. Malreduction can lead to lateral rotation of the talus, tipping of the mortise, and widening of the medial clear space [20]. Changes in joint contact area can be dramatically altered with a small lateral shift of the talus. Ramsey and Hamilton [21] reported a 42% decrease in joint contact area with a 1-mm lateral shift of the talus. Other studies have demonstrated changes in joint contact pressures with displacement of ankle fractures [22–24]. Valgus malunion can lead to similar changes. Concern for malunion is higher in patients who have a history of comminution at the fracture site at the time of injury. Accurate length, alignment, and rotation of the fibula are critical to normal ankle function. In addition to malalignment, malunion of the fibula can lead to syndesmotic instability and apparent widening of the mortise on routine radiographs. This result is often subtle and comparison to the contralateral extremity can be beneficial. Overlap of the distal tibia and fibula at the syndesmosis may still be present but asymmetric on comparison mortise views. This finding can range from obvious to only apparent with scrutiny. Flexion malunion can shift the lateral malleolus posterior in the incisura leading to widening, whereas extension malunions can lead to an anterior shift in the incisura and widening. Deformities can be multiplanar. Patients tend to present with complaints of persistent swelling and complaints of worsening pain with activity. Many feel the ankle has "never been right" since the time of injury. Evaluation should consist of a standard physical examination of the foot and ankle. Competency of the lateral ankle ligaments and deltoid should be thoroughly evaluated. Radiographic examination includes anteroposterior, lateral, and mortise images. Contralateral images are ordered as needed. The relationship between the lateral gutter of the ankle mortise and the subfibular recess should be evaluated. CT imaging is often helpful to evaluate the relationship of the lateral malleolus to the incisura fibularis with greater detail.

Surgical treatment

The patient is placed supine and a bump is placed under the ipsilateral hip. Images of the contralateral mortise and lateral are obtained using fluoroscopy, printed, and taped to the bottom of the monitor to allow rapid comparison. Retained hardware, if present, is removed. If the syndesmosis is not congruent because of widening or translation of the fibula either anterior or posterior, dissection is carried over the front of the fibula and into the syndesmosis. Typically a large amount of fibrous scar tissue is present and must be resected to allow the distal end of the fibula to move. The type of osteotomy depends on the malunion present. Transverse osteotomies have been described and are best for pure rotation malalignment [25]. If the deformity is shortening, a longitudinal osteotomy can obtain length by sliding the distal fibula. Anterior or posterior malalignment can be addressed. Multiplanar deformities are best addressed by oblique osteotomies. Fixation techniques vary according to available bone stock, bone density, and holes from prior fixation. Rigid fixation is necessary to optimize healing. If fixation was present laterally on the fibula the new fixation can be applied posteriorly to allow screw trajectory in a different plane (Fig. 2). Location of the lateral malleolus to the subfibular recess and lateral process are evaluated on the mortise along with tibia–fibula overlap. Medial clear space should no longer be increased and the mortise should be congruent when the reduction is correct. None of the osteotomy fixation should be inserted across the syndesmosis. After the osteotomy is completed and rigidly fixed, competency of the syndesmosis is assessed. If unstable or incongruent, a large reduction clamp is used to reduce the fibula back into the correct position in the

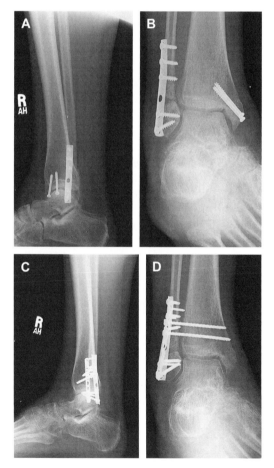

Fig. 2. This patient is a 26-year-old man who sustained a bimalleolar ankle fracture as a result of a motorcycle accident. (A, B) Preoperative images show a short and malpositioned fibula with syndesmotic widening. There is questionable union of the lateral malleolus fracture. (C, D) Postoperative images show fibular length to be restored and syndesmotic relationship to be re-established.

incisura fibularis. If posterior or anterior displacement is present they are corrected. Direct visualization is helpful. Additionally the distance from the posterior cortex of the fibula to the posterior cortex of the tibia at the joint level on a radiograph can be compared with the contralateral images. Once correct, two Kirschner wires are used as provisional fixation to hold reduction while screws are inserted. Bone graft, if needed, is obtained from the ipsilateral calcaneus or proximal tibia. Postoperatively the patient is placed in a splint and restricted to non–weight-bearing for 6 to 8 weeks until union occurs.

Results

Results for fibular osteotomies for arthritic changes in the ankle are variable. Marti and colleagues [20] reported on osteotomies for malunion of ankle fractures in 31 patients. Six had radiographic evidence of arthritis preoperatively with no progression of arthritis appreciated at final follow-up. Interval between injury and reconstruction and age were not factors. Severe arthritis led to worse results. He concluded that reconstruction should be the first step in treating arthritis as a result of malunion. Arthrodesis and supramalleolar osteotomy should be reserved for patients who fail correction of the fibula malunion. Marti also concluded that arthritic changes were better tolerated once alignment was restored. Hughes [26] reported on 28 patients treated with lengthening fibular osteotomies and bone graft. Incongruent mortise, lateral shift of the talus, and a shortened fibula were common. A total of 22 patients had good or excellent outcomes. No difference was seen in outcome with age or interval from injury. Weber and Simpson [27] reported on 23 cases of fibular lengthening osteotomies to correct malunion. A total of 17 had good or excellent results, whereas 6 had poor results. The poor results were seen in patients who radiographically had moderate to severe arthritis before surgical correction. The authors believed there was no time limit on the procedure but recommended arthrodesis for patients who had severe degenerative changes.

Hindfoot and midfoot osteotomy for ankle arthritis

Results of osteotomies on the hindfoot and midfoot for ankle arthritis have not been reviewed in any long-term study. Research has demonstrated that alterations in alignment about the ankle have significant effects on articular surfaces [28]. This approach to ankle arthritis can be used in patients who are not ideal for more definitive procedures for ankle arthritis. Young age at the time of arthrodesis can lead to arthritic changes in other joints of the foot [29]. Total ankle arthroplasty is not ideally suited for the young patient at this time and is better suited for older patients [30,31]. These procedures can be used as an attempt to buy time before other procedures, including arthrodesis and arthroplasty, are required. Osteotomies of the ankle and hindfoot can also be of benefit in patients who have arthritis as a result of long-standing lateral ankle instability (Fig. 3). Excessive forefoot or hindfoot varus can also lead to varus tipping and ankle arthritis. By history it is occasionally difficult to determine which came first, the lateral ankle instability or the varus deformity. Both instability and hindfoot varus may be a result of an underlying cavus foot deformity. The cavus may be quite obvious or very subtle. Hindfoot deformities occasionally present with initial complaints of ankle pain from arthritis. Years of ambulation on the outside of the foot can lead to laxity of the lateral ankle ligaments. The instability patients often provide a history of more than 20 years of instability. Many can recall their first episode of instability.

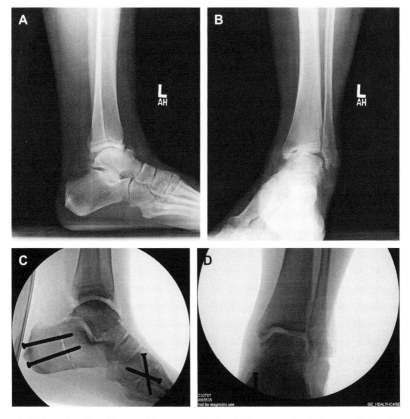

Fig. 3. This patient is a 55-year-old woman who has had greater than 25 years of ankle instability. (A, B) Preoperative images demonstrate anterior ankle impingement on the lateral and severe varus tipping on the mortise image. (C, D) The patient was treated operatively with a lateralizing calcaneal osteotomy, dorsiflexion osteotomy at the first tarsometatarsal joint, lateral ankle reconstruction, and ankle arthrotomy and cheilectomy, with significant improvement of the ankle alignment.

Physical examination

Physical examination should consist of a thorough examination of the lower leg, foot, and ankle. Overall alignment of the lower extremity should be evaluated. Standing examination consists of observation of the alignment of the foot and ankle while standing both from behind and from in front of the patient. Hindfoot alignment should be examined carefully for varus. When observed from the front the medial aspect of the foot should be observed to see if a small portion of the heel is visible. With normal hindfoot valgus it is not possible to see the heel along the medial aspect of the foot. If present this is considered a peekaboo heel sign and is consistent with varus [32]. The presence of callosities on the lateral portion of the foot may also result from varus. Forefoot varus can contribute to the overall foot deformity leading to ankle arthritis. The first ray should be carefully examined. This ray can either be plantar flexed in rigid fashion through the first tarsometatarsal joint or may be a dynamically plantar flexed first ray from peroneus longus overdrive. The forefoot should be examined with the patient seated. The forefoot should be relatively balanced and even when looking across the metatarsal heads. If the first ray is rigidly plantar flexed it will be lower than the other metatarsal heads. By assessing the motor strength and function of the peroneus longus it is possible to determine its role in the overall varus. A Coleman block is also a useful examination aid. If the patient stands on the Coleman block with the first ray dropped off the block and the hindfoot alignment corrects, the varus is forefoot driven. Competency of the lateral ankle ligaments and deltoid should be examined by anterior drawer and talar tilt and compared with the contralateral. Radiographic review should consist of standing mortise, lateral foot, and ankle images. Tipping of the talus in the mortise, anterior osteophytes off the distal tibia and talar neck, subchondral sclerosis, and cystic changes are findings consistent with arthritis. The orientation of the first metatarsal is steeper relative to the floor in patients who have forefoot varus. The metatarsals may also appear stacked, with minimal overlap of one metatarsal over the other on the lateral standing image. All patients should be evaluated for equinus contracture. Passive range of motion should be assessed first because dorsiflexion is often limited by anterior osteophytes in the arthritic population. Ankle dorsiflexion is measured with the talonavicular joint held in neutral. Range of motion is evaluated with the knee extended and flexed. Gastrocnemius equinus exists if the ankle does not dorsiflex past neutral with the knee extended, but can dorsiflex beyond neutral with the knee flexed. If knee flexion does not improve the ability to dorsiflex at the ankle the equinus is fixed and is the result of Achilles contracture. These examination findings are important and should be evaluated routinely as part of any presurgical work-up. In patients who have anterior osteophytes present, equinus should be evaluated in the operative suite after the osteophytes have been addressed.

Surgical treatment

Surgical treatment varies depending on the results of the clinical examination. The goal of the surgical reconstruction is to rebalance the foot such that with weight-bearing the ankle does not tip into varus. This procedure theoretically distributes the contact forces onto a broader surface area of articular cartilage and onto areas that are less arthritic. The patient is positioned supine on the operative table so that the feet are at the very end of the table to facilitate placement of hardware. The first tarsometatarsal joint is approached and débrided of all cartilage. Using a saw a dorsally based wedge is removed from the first metatarsal, including the articular surface. The metatarsal is then dorsiflexed to correct the deformity and rigidly fixed with two 4.0-mm screws. Care is taken to avoid taking bone from the plantar cortex to avoid shortening. A large amount of correction can be achieved by removing a small amount of bone because of the proximal location of this osteotomy. Dissection is then carried down to the lateral aspect of the calcaneus behind the sural nerve and peroneal tendons. Using a saw an osteotomy is created with a saw blade. The osteotomy must be made so that the Achilles, articular surface of the posterior facet, and the origin of the plantar fascia are left preserved. Care is taken to prevent injury to the medial neurovascular and tendinous structures as the medial cortex is cut. The heel is then shifted laterally 0.5 to 1 cm, depending on the case, and held provisionally with Kirschner wires. The osteotomy is secured with 6.5-mm or 4-mm screws. Next a curvilinear incision is made behind and around the distal fibula. If the anterior talofibular ligament and calcaneofibular ligament are present they can be reconstructed as a modified Broström-type repair. Alternatively, a reconstruction using a portion of tendon can be used. The peroneal tendons can be examined around the fibula to assess for any tears or frank rupture. If the long peroneal tendon contributes to the varus, it can be transferred into peroneus brevis above the lateral malleolus through the same incision. This procedure weakens the role of the peroneus longus and its contribution to varus and provides more strength to eversion. Equinus, if present, is addressed by a tendo Achilles lengthening or a gastrocnemius recession. Patients are immobilized after surgery and are typically non–weight-bearing for 6 to 8 weeks until radiographic evidence of healing.

Similar procedures may be used to treat valgus ankle arthritis if it is deemed to be secondary to foot malalignment. The calcaneal osteotomy can be performed and slid medial, the first ray plantar flexed by osteotomy at the first tarsometatarsal, and other pathology addressed. Careful assessment of tibialis posterior function is necessary in valgus malalignment and its role is beyond the scope of this article.

No long-term studies for combined hindfoot and midfoot osteotomies for the treatment of ankle arthritis have been reported.

Summary

Ankle arthrodesis continues to be the procedure of choice for ankle arthritis. Coester and colleagues [29] showed that arthrodesis is a significant risk factor for development of arthritis in the ipsilateral hindfoot and forefoot, however. Total ankle arthroplasty has gained significant interest but is not yet ideally suited for younger active patients because of unacceptable failure rates and complications [30,31]. Osteotomies can play an important role in re-establishing normal alignment and potentially decreasing the rate of progression of wear on the articular surfaces and decreasing pain, which may allow more time before arthrodesis or arthroplasty are needed. The success of total ankle arthroplasty depends largely on the alignment of the foot and ankle and osteotomies can be used in a staged manner as part of a reconstructive effort including total ankle arthroplasty. Supramalleolar osteotomies can be used to align the tibia; alternatively, osteotomies in the midfoot and hindfoot can be used to balance the foot and ankle making them suitable for arthroplasty in an individual who perhaps would not otherwise have that treatment option. Further studies will continue to clarify the role and indications for osteotomies for treatment of ankle arthritis.

References

[1] Abraham E, Lubicky JP, Songer MN, et al. Supramalleolar osteotomy for ankle valgus in myelomeningocele. J Pediatr Orthop 1996;16:774–81.

[2] Dodgin DA, De Swart RJ, Stefko RM, et al. Distal tibial/fibular derotation osteotomy for correction of tibial torsion: review of technique and results in 63 cases. J Pediatr Orthop 1998;18:95–101.

[3] Fraser RK, Menelaus MB. The management of tibial torsion in patients with spinal bifida. J Bone Joint Surg Br 1993;75:495–7.

[4] Kumar SJ, Keret D, MacEWenm DG. Corrective cosmetic supramalleolar for valgus deformity of the ankle joint: a report of two cases. J Pediatr Orthop 1990;10A:124–7.

[5] Malhorta D, Puri R, Owen R. Valgus deformity of the ankle in children with spina bifida aperta. J Bone Joint Surg Br 1984;66:381–5.

[6] Lubicky JP, Altiok H. Transphyseal osteotomy of the distal tibia for correction of valgus/varus deformities of the ankle. J Pediatr Orthop 2001;21A:80–8.

[7] Merchant TC, Dietz FR. Long-term follow-up after fractures of the tibial and fibular shafts. J Bone Joint Surg Am 1989;71:599–606.

[8] Puno RM, Vaughan JJ, Stretten ML, et al. Long-term effects of tibial angular malunion on the knee and ankle joints. J Orthop Trauma 1991;5:247–54.

[9] Milner SA, Davis TR, Muir KR, et al. Long-term outcome after tibial shaft fracture: is malunion important? J Bone Joint Surg Am 2002;84:971–80.

[10] Ting AJ, Tarr RR, Sarmeinto A, et al. The role of subtalar motion and ankle contact pressure changes from angular deformities of the tibia. Foot Ankle 1987;7:290–9.

[11] Tarr RR, Resnick CT, Wagner KS, et al. Changes in tibiotalar joint contact areas following experimentally induced tibial angular deformity. Clin Orthop 1985;199:72–80.

[12] Takakura Y, Tanaka Y, Kumai T, et al. Low tibial osteotomy for osteoarthritis of the ankle. Results of a new operation in 18 patients. J Bone Joint Surg 1995;77(1):50–4.

[13] Stamatis ED, Cooper PS, Myerson MS. Supramalleolar osteotomy for the treatment of distal tibia angular deformities and arthritis of the ankle joint. Foot Ankle Int 2003; 24(10):754–64.

[14] Avecedo JI, Myerson MS. Reconstructive alternatives for ankle arthritis. Foot Ankle Clin 1999;4:409–30.
[15] Takakura Y, et al. The treatment for osteoarthritis of the ankle joint. Jpn J Rheum Joint Surg 1986;5:347–52.
[16] Sangeorzan BJ, Sangeorzan BP, Hansen ST, et al. Mathematically directed single-cut osteotomy for correction of tibial malunion. J Orthop Trauma 1989;3:267–75.
[17] Takakura Y, Takaoka T, Tanaka Y, et al. Result of opening-wedge osteotomy for the treatment of a post-traumatic varus deformity of the ankle. J Bone Joint Surg Am 1998;80:213–8.
[18] Weber BG. Die Verletzungen des oberen Sprunggelenkes. 2 Aufl. Bern (Switzerland): Verlag Hans Huber; 1972 [in German].
[19] Yablon IG, Heller FG, Shouse L. The key role of the lateral malleolus in displaced fractures of the ankle. J Bone Joint Surg Am 1977;59:169–73.
[20] Marti RK, Raaymakers ELFB, Nolte PA. Malunited ankle fractures the late results of reconstruction. J Bone Joint Surg Br 1990;72:709–13.
[21] Ramsey P, Hamilton W. Changes in tibiotalar area of contact caused by lateral talar tilt shift. J Bone Joint Surg Am 1976;58:356–7.
[22] Burns WC, Prakash K, Adalaar RS, et al. Tibiotalar joint dynamics: indications for the syndesmotic screw. A cadaver study. Foot Ankle 1993;14:153–8.
[23] Macko VM, Matthews LS, Zwerkoski P, et al. The joint contact area of the ankle. The contribution of the posterior malleolus. J Bone Joint Surg Am 1991;73:347–51.
[24] Vrahas M, Fu F, Veenis B, et al. Intra-articular contact stress with simulated ankle malunions. J Orthop Trauma 1994;8(2):159–66.
[25] Austin RT. Rotatory malunion of the lateral malleolus corrected by osteotomy. J Bone Joint Surg Br 1987;69:481.
[26] Hughes JL. Corrective osteotomies of the fibula after defectively healed ankle fractures. J Bone Joint Surg Am 1976;58:728.
[27] Weber BG, Simpson LA. Corrective lengthening osteotomy of the fibula. Clin Orthop 1985; 199:61–7.
[28] Steffensmeier SJ, Berbaum KS, Brown TD. Effects of medial and lateral displacement calcaneal osteotomies on tibiotalar joint contact stresses. J Orthop Res 1996;14(6):980–5.
[29] Coester LM, Saltzman CL, Leupold J. Long-term results following ankle arthrodesis for post-traumatic arthritis. J Bone Joint Surg Am 2001;83(2):219–28.
[30] Pyevich MT, Saltzman CL, Callaghan JJ, et al. Total ankle arthroplasty: a unique design. Two to twelve year follow up. J Bone Joint Surg Am 1998;80(10):1410–20.
[31] Spirt AA, Assal M, Hansen ST. Complications and failure after total ankle arthroplasty. J Bone Joint Surg Am 2004;86(6):11720–8.
[32] Manoli A, Graham B. The subtle cavus foot "the underpronator". Foot Ankle Int 2005; 26(3):256–63.

ELSEVIER
SAUNDERS

Foot Ankle Clin N Am
12 (2007) 15–27

FOOT AND
ANKLE CLINICS

The Valgus Ankle

Vic Gibson, DO[a],*, David Prieskorn, DO[b]

[a]Orthopedic surgery resident, Botsford General Hospital, 28050 Grand River,
Farmington Hills, MI 48336, USA
[b]Tri County Orthopedics, 28100 Grand River, Suite 209, Farmington Hills, MI 48336, USA

The valgus ankle is a complex deformity with many possible origins. The most common cause, however, is degenerative in the form of untreated chronic posterior tibial tendon dysfunction. Regardless of the cause, the principles of treatment remain the same: one must attempt to achieve a painless, plantigrade foot while preserving maximal flexibility. Various options are available for treatment, including osteotomies, fusions, and arthroplasty. Each has its own advantages and disadvantages. The valgus ankle can lead to severe deformity, debility, and pain, stressing the importance of optimal management of this condition (Fig. 1). This article reviews the entity of the valgus ankle, discusses its clinical recognition, and reviews forms of treatment.

Anatomy

The anatomy of the valgus ankle is important to understand, particularly the medial structures that help stabilize the ankle joint. The ankle joint is a complex hinge joint, which has articulations between the tibia, fibula, and talus, supported by a complex ligamentous system. The lateral malleolus, along with the lateral collateral ligaments, help provide lateral support to the ankle. The syndesmotic ligament complex provides stability between the distal fibula and tibia to maintain the structural integrity of the mortise. The medial malleolus articulates with the medial facet of the talus and is divided into the anterior and posterior colliculus, which serves as attachments for the deltoid ligament.

The deltoid ligament provides the medial ligamentous support. The deltoid is divided into the superficial and deep components. The superficial

* Corresponding author.
E-mail address: ggibson@botsford.org (V. Gibson).

1083-7515/07/$ - see front matter
doi:10.1016/j.fcl.2006.11.001

foot.theclinics.com

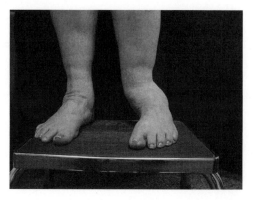

Fig. 1. Severe deformity caused by a valgus ankle.

deltoid was described as having five fascicles based on their insertions [1–3]. The anterior superficial tibiotalar fascicle originates from the anterior border of the anterior colliculus and inserts along the dorsal portion of the talar neck proximal to the talonavicular capsule. The tibionavicular fascicle takes its origin from the anterior colliculus and inserts on the navicular. The tibioligamentous fascicle originates from the anterior colliculus and inserts on the superior border of the superomedial calcaneonavicular ligament. These three anterior fascicles of the superficial deltoid ligament are more broad but weaker than the other components. The fourth fascicle, the tibiocalcaneal fascicle, is the strongest component of the superficial deltoid ligament and crosses the ankle and subtalar joint. It originates from the medial aspect of the anterior colliculus and inserts onto the sustentaculum tali, merging with the superomedial calcaneonavicular ligament. Injury to this fascicle was reported to have the largest effect on tibiotalar contact pressures than injury to any of the other fascicles [4,5]. The posterior superficial tibiotalar fascicle originates from the posterior medial surface of the anterior colliculus and inserts on the posterior medial tibiotalar tubercle.

The deep deltoid ligament is a short and strong ligament and consists of two components. The anterior tibiotalar ligament originates from the anterior colliculus and inserts on the medial talus. The posterior tibiotalar ligament originates from the posterior surface of the anterior colliculus, the intercollicular fossa, and anterior aspect of the posterior colliculus. It is the strongest component of the deltoid and functions as a medial and posterior stabilizer.

Pathogenesis

The pathogenesis is determined by the origin of the valgus ankle. Several conditions can result in a valgus ankle deformity. These include developmental causes (eg, fibular hemimelia), cartilage injuries (eg, post-traumatic arthrosis, lateral osteochondral defects), and ligamentous imbalance (eg, posterior tibial tendon deficiency [PTTD], deltoid ligament injury). The most common cause of this deformity is end-stage PTTD.

Johnson and Strom [6] were the first to describe three clinical stages of PTTD. Stage I is tendonitis of the posterior tibial tendon without deformity. Stage II tendon insufficiency results in tendon elongation with a flexible hindfoot valgus deformity. The elongation of the tendon may be precipitated by a traumatic tear (Fig. 2) or may be degenerative. Stage III insufficiency results in a rigid hindfoot valgus deformity. Although Johnson and Strom alluded to a probable stage IV in 1989, Myerson is credited with the first description of stage IV disease, which is described as a fixed hindfoot valgus deformity producing a valgus talar tilt [6,12]. Since that time however, published literature has been deficient in describing treatment options and long-term outcome related to stage IV PTTD.

In the case of stage IV PTTD, the hindfoot valgus causes attrition of the tibiocalcaneal fascicle, tibioligamentous fascicle, and the spring ligament complex [1,2]. This leaves the deep deltoid ligament as the only restraint to a tilted ankle. Cadaver studies have shown the importance of both the superficial and deep components as a restraint to talar tilt [4,7]. When only one component was sectioned, no tilt was observed; only after both superficial and deep components were sectioned was significant talar tilt observed. With a long-standing hindfoot valgus, the Achilles tendon is displaced lateral to the subtalar joint and the gastrocnemius–soleus complex becomes contracted [8,9]. This action continues to change the mechanical axis of the lower extremity, concentrating the weight-bearing tension load on the medial supporting structures, and could lead to attrition and elongation of the deltoid ligament and valgus tilting of the ankle as the deformity

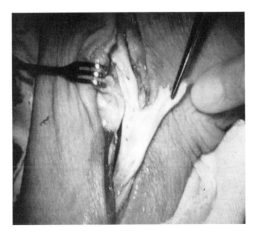

Fig. 2. A traumatic partial tear of the posterior tibial tendon.

increases. Cadaver studies have shown that after sectioning the superficial deltoid ligament, contact areas were significantly reduced and peak pressures significantly increased, emphasizing the stress placed on the tibiotalar joint that may be responsible for degenerative changes that can occur with a long-term deformity [4,5].

Stage IV disease can occur after triple arthrodesis for stage III PTTD (Fig. 3). Triple arthrodesis is commonly used for stage III PTTD with a fixed deformity or arthrosis in the subtalar, talonavicular, and calcaneocuboid joints. Residual hindfoot valgus post–triple arthrodesis leads to increased deltoid ligament strain through translational forces across the ankle. Further attenuation or failure of the deltoid ligament leads to a valgus tilt of the talus. Cadaver studies have shown that residual hindfoot valgus after triple arthrodesis showed a 76% increase in deltoid ligament strain [17].

Clinical examination

The foot and ankle examination should always begin with obtaining an adequate history. Patients who have PTTD usually report an insidious onset [2,8,9]. In stage I of the disease, patients usually complain of pain and swelling over the medial aspect of the foot. The tendon retains function and is capable of a single-foot toe raise with medial pain. In stage II, the longitudinal arch of the foot shows collapse. Medial wear of the shoe occurs and a single toe raise is no longer possible on the affected side. Manual testing still shows a well-defined tendon. It will be painful to touch and often is inflamed posterior and inferior to the medial malleolus. As the deformity progresses to stage III, hindfoot valgus becomes more prominent and the

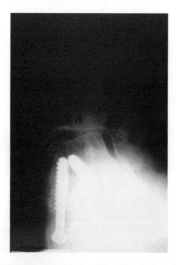

Fig. 3. Anteroposterior radiograph showing a valgus tilt of the talus after a triple arthrodesis.

individual can no longer independently contract the posterior tibial tendon against resistance. Early in stage III the subtalar joint is still flexible to passive range of motion, making it amendable to tendon transfer [1,11]. Later the joint becomes fixed in a valgus posture, making corrective arthrodesis the only viable option. Pain can occur along the lateral aspect of the foot secondary to impingement between the calcaneus and fibula.

Physical examination of the foot and ankle should start by evaluating the overall alignment of both lower extremities. Any knee or tibia deformity can accentuate a valgus hindfoot [2]. The anterior view of stage II through IV PTTD shows a prominent medial border of the foot and a collapsed longitudinal arch. Posteriorly the hindfoot will be in valgus and have the "too many toes" sign. During the heel rise test, the hindfoot will remain in an everted position. The subtalar and transverse tarsal joint motion should be assessed. Contracture of the gastrocnemius and peroneal tendons occurs in a long-standing deformity. The ankle may be tender to palpation in a flexible or fixed deformity. The clinical examination of stage III and stage IV are very similar, and therefore stage IV may best be seen on anteroposterior radiographs as valgus tilting of the talar dome.

Radiographs are important in assessing a patient's condition. Appropriate radiographs include standing anteroposterior views of both ankles and standing anteroposterior, Harris, and lateral views of both feet. Valgus tilting of the talus is diagnosed on the anteroposterior view of the ankle. A mortise view may also be helpful to assess chondral compression in the lateral gutter and lateral talar dome. Talar tilt is defined as a difference between the medial and lateral ankle clear space greater than 2 mm, and indicates a likely deltoid ligament injury (Fig. 4) [1]. Other findings include arthritic

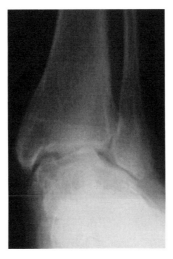

Fig. 4. Anteroposterior radiograph showing valgus tilt of the ankle in the mortise.

changes with osteophytes, sclerosis, and subchondral cyst formation. Stress radiographs may help determine the reducibility of the ankle mortise.

Management

Nonoperative

The initial management of all stages of PTTD should begin with a trial of conservative treatment [8,9]. Rest, nonsteroidal anti-inflammatory drugs, activity modification, and use of orthotics are the mainstays of conservative therapy. Immobilization with an orthotic device can be used to provide pain relief, retard progression, and accommodate a fixed deformity. In a fixed deformity, the orthosis must be accommodative rather than corrective, because the latter can increase pain and cause skin breakdown (Fig. 5). Options for orthoses include the University of California Biomechanics Laboratory brace, ankle foot orthosis, Arizona brace, or Marzano-style brace. At this stage of the disease, however, conservative management is difficult, rarely leads to a successful outcome, and is indicated in patients who have comorbidities that prevent surgical options [1].

The goals of surgery are to maximize flexibility and produce a painless and plantigrade foot without the need for supplementary bracing. Ankle, hindfoot, and midfoot flexibility cannot always be restored. Multiple options are often available for correction, but no clinical studies show which options are clearly superior. These options include distal malleolar osteotomy, tibiotalocalcaneal fusion, and pantalar fusion, or ankle arthroplasty with or without supplemental hindfoot corrective surgery.

Tibiotalocalcaneal arthrodesis

Tibiotalocalcaneal arthrodesis involves fusion of the ankle and subtalar joints. This procedure can be performed if the talonavicular and

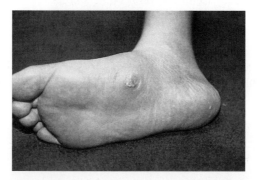

Fig. 5. Skin breakdown in a patient who had a fixed deformity treated with corrective orthosis.

calcaneocuboid joints are spared. The ankle should be maintained at neutral to 10° of dorsiflexion to improve transfer of weight from heel strike to mid-stance phase of gait. The subtalar joint should be fused at 5° of valgus to maintain flexibility of the midfoot. A tibiotalocalcaneal fusion can be obtained through external fixation, internal fixation, or retrograde intramedullary nailing [13–16]. Chou and colleagues [15] reported on tibiotalocalcaneal arthrodesis in 55 patients with average follow-up of 28 months. Union was achieved in 48 ankles with an average time of 19 weeks, and 40 patients required a shoe modification or orthosis, indicating the need for supplementary management after this type of procedure. Even with supplementary modification, 48 patients (87%) reported a satisfactory result. Patients who underwent a tibiotalocalcaneal fusion were more mobile and function at a higher level than the pantalar group [10].

Technique

After a spinal or general anesthetic is administered, patients are placed in a supine position with a lateral bump to control external rotation of the limb. Care is taken to examine the opposite extremity and replicate the amount of rotation identified in the normal limb. The approach is lateral, beginning 6 cm proximal to the distal fibula, and curves inferior to the lateral aspect of the calcaneal cuboid joint. The distal 3 to 4 cm of the fibula is resected and morselized to be used as bone graft. A subperiosteal dissection is performed anterior and posterior to the ankle joint to allow visualization of the subtalar and tibiotalar joints.

The architecture and circulation of the talus are assessed. If the talus is salvageable, both the tibiotalar and talar calcaneal joints are denuded of all articular cartilage. Care is taken to not break off the medial malleolus on the medial aspect of the ankle. If the talus is salvageable, retaining it is always best to maintain relatively normal length of the limb. A second incision on the medial aspect of the ankle measuring 3 cm from the tip of the medial malleolus distalward may be performed to allow visualization of the articular surface of the medial malleolus. A ribbon retractor can be placed between neurovascular structures and the posterior aspect of the ankle joint through this incision.

All three facets of the subtalar joint are denuded of cartilage and the foot is held in proper orientation to all three planes. The alignment is compared with the opposite limb. A third incision is made on the plantar aspect of the foot 3 cm in length and aligned with the tibial axis. This incision is longitudinally oriented using blunt dissection down to the inferior aspect of the calcaneus. Neurovascular structures on the plantar aspect of the foot are protected by a tissue protector and a guidewire is placed 1 cm anterior and 1 cm medial to the tuberosity of the calcaneus. Using sequential flexible reamers, the tibial canal, talar body, and calcaneus are prepared for fixation. After the rod is inserted, locking screws are applied to the tibia and calcaneus. The authors prefer a rod, which provides compression across the joint to encourage osteogenesis at the arthrodesis locations. A layered closure is performed and radiographs taken to provide proper location and orientation of the limb at that time.

Pantalar arthrodesis

Pantalar arthrodesis involves fusion of the subtalar, talonavicular, calcaneocuboid, and tibiotalar joints. This procedure remains an option for patients who have degenerative changes involving these joints. Realignment is possible in most cases, but loss of motion in all three planes can be devastating to patients. Patients must be advised that the limited mobility and stiffness after this type of procedure is intolerant of shoe wear and will increase the likelihood of knee and hip arthrosis [16]. This procedure is technically difficult, but provides an alternative to amputation and may improve quality of life in patients who have severe deformities [16]. Several studies have shown good fusion rates and pain relief for pantalar arthrodesis in patients who have poliomyelitis, myelodysplasia, rheumatoid arthritis, and post-traumatic arthrosis and deformity [18–21].

Technique

After a spinal or general anesthetic is administered, patients are placed in a supine position with a lateral bump to control external rotation of the limb. The fusion of the talonavicular and calcaneocuboid joints can be achieved using an intramedullary rod. An alternative involves fixation screws entering the posterior aspect of the calcaneal tuberosity through the talus, with purchase obtained in the anterior cortex of the distal tibia. A pediatric blade plate can also be used to provide fixation through the lateral approach.

Satisfactory positioning in all three planes, including compression of the tibiotalar and talocalcaneal joints, must be assured. Attention can then be directed to the talonavicular arthrodesis. The medial incision begins one centimeter distal to the medial malleolus and courses along the navicular to the medial aspect of the first cuneiform. The incision is taken down subperiosteally with dissection dorsal and plantar over the talonavicular joint. Using a curved osteotome, curet, and rongeur, the articular surface is then denuded of cartilage. Subchondral bone must not be denuded to promote optimal contact before fixation. Poor contact often indicates a poor reduction. The surface area of the respective bones can be increased by feathering with the quarter-inch osteotome. A fracture of this cortex will affect the purchase of the 4.0 mm cancellous screws.

Before compressing this joint, attention is directed to the calcaneal cuboid joint. This incision is directly lateral and extends 3 cm centered over the calcaneal cuboid joint. Using curved and straight osteotomes, the articular surfaces are again denuded of cartilage and the surface area is increased using a quarter-inch osteotome. The articular surfaces are then held in proper position, correcting any forefoot varus that may have resulted from a chronic valgus ankle deformity.

Fixation is first obtained laterally in the calcaneal cuboid joint with either crossing screws or staples. Once the lateral aspect of the mid-foot is secure, both joints are compressed through tightening of the medial cancellous screws. As the screws tighten, the navicular should approximate the denuded talar head similar to a closing book, providing maximal contact and stability. A layered closure of all incisions is then performed.

Distal malleolar osteotomy

Distal malleolar osteotomies have been used with good results for pediatric patients, and experts have recently shown interest in using them in adult populations. Indications for supramalleolar osteotomy for reconstruction of the adult hindfoot include:

1) Angular correction for ankle joint osteoarthritis
2) Correction of distal tibial malunion
3) Correction of lower-extremity malalignment as a staging procedure for total ankle arthroplasty
4) Correction of malunion after ankle arthrodesis
5) Correction of ankle valgus in cases of ball and socket ankle that result from extensive tarsal coalition
6) Correction of hindfoot malalignment in cases of neuroarthropathy or distal tibial avascular necrosis [22]

A successful outcome requires careful attention to several "osteotomy rules." Bone deformity must be planned by drawing axis lines for each joint segment and diaphysial segment. Fixation methods may include plates and screws for uniplanar correction or external fixators if multiplanar correction is required [22–27].

If PTTD 4 is the cause of the deformity, attention must also be directed to hindfoot support. The choice of flexor digitorum longus– or flexor hallucis longus–tendon transfer with or without osteotomy, or hindfoot fusion is made according to the condition of the subtalar joint [11,28].

Total ankle arthroplasty

The role of total ankle replacement (TAR) in treating a valgus ankle has not clearly been defined. The ideal patient is older, usually older than 60 years, with low functional demands and arthrosis of the ankle or other hindfoot joints [29–31]. Patients who have severe malalignment may require staged procedures to correct the malalignment before a TAR can be performed [21,27,30]. The goal of TAR is to achieve a normal range of motion using a stable prosthesis within the constraints of the ligamentous complex of the ankle.

Technique

The patient is placed in a supine position with a sandbag placed under the affected side. A thigh tourniquet is used for homeostasis. A bone distractor is placed on the medial aspect of the ankle not only to distract the ankle joint but also to correct either the valgus or varus malalignment before the tibial and talar osteotomies. A longitudinal anterior incision is deepened between the extensor hallucis longus and anterior tibial tendons. The superficial peroneal nerve is identified and retracted laterally. The anterior ankle capsule is incised longitudinally and the medial, anterior, and lateral tibia are subperiosteally exposed. The anterior osteophytes are resected along the border of the talus. A longitudinal incision is made along the anterior border of the distal fibula. The anterior tibiofibular ligament is excised and the syndesmosis is mobilized with an osteotome. The lateral malleolus can be released laterally, but care must be taken to avoid fracture of the fibula.

The TAR alignment guide is centered just distal to the tibial tubercule in line with the axis of the tibia. The cutting block is centered over the ankle joint. Care must be taken to avoid removing excessive medial bone from the medial malleolus or excessive bone from the lateral malleolus. An oscillating saw is used to create osteotomies in the distal tibia, with the syndesmosis carefully protected. At the medial osteotomy, care must be taken to avoid fracturing the medial malleolus. A reciprocating saw is used to complete the cuts in the corner of the tibia. The tibial bone may be sectioned to remove the bone piecemeal. The dome of the talus is osteotomized, with care taken to avoid injury to the neurovascular bundle on the posteromedial aspect of the ankle. Dense talar bone may make this osteotomy difficult. A symmetric cut is most important.

Tibial trial components are placed based on the preoperative templating. During the insertion of the tibial component, the syndesmosis is distracted with an osteotome. A small V cut is made in an anteroposterior direction in the distal tibial plafond region to secure the position of the tibial component. A trial insert is then impacted into place in an anteroposterior direction and is driven until it is flush against the medial and lateral malleolus. A trough is cut in the talus in line with the body of the talus (not the neck of the talus). A trial talar component is driven in an anteroposterior direction until it is well seated. The components are inspected for fit, range of motion, and stability.

Surgeons must decide at this point whether to cement the components or use biologic fixation. If biologic fixation is chosen, the tibial component is impacted into place. Some upward pressure may be necessary to seat the component. The component is impacted until the prosthesis is flush with the anterior tibial cortex. The talar component is then impacted into place until the talar dome drops inside the anterior lip of the polyethylene on the tibial component. The talar component must not be driven too far posteriorly. Because in the presence of significant arthritis the talus is often

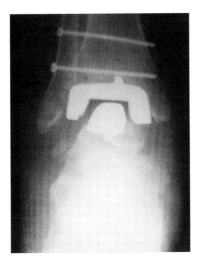

Fig. 6. Anteroposterior radiograph showing acceptable position of the components of a total ankle replacement.

subluxed anteriorly, care must be taken to avoid posterior translation of the talar component. Additional distraction may be necessary to seat the talar component.

The ankle distractor is then removed. Intraoperative radiographs or fluoroscopy may be used to visualize the position of the components (Fig. 6). Range of motion of the ankle is inspected. Motion may vary depending on the length of immobility and the amount of preoperative fibrosis. Through a lateral incision, the tibiofibular syndesmosis is decorticated and feathered with a small osteotome. Morselized bone that has been resected from the tibial and talar region is placed into this interval. Two cross-syndesmotic screws are placed to stabilize the syndesmosis. The anterior and lateral wounds are closed in a routine and layered manner. Meticulous closure is important, with separate closure of the fascia, subcutaneous tissue, and skin.

Summary

When a deformity of the hindfoot advances to the point where it begins to affect the alignment of the ankle, it becomes a particularly challenging problem to correct. Nonoperative options are limited and should be reserved for patients who have comorbidities prohibiting surgical attention. The associated deformities must first be corrected to protect the ankle realignment procedure. The goals of treatment are to maximize flexibility and produce a painless and plantigrade foot without the need for supplementary bracing.

References

[1] Kelly IP, Nunley JA. Treatment of stage 4 adult acquired flat foot. Foot Ankle Clin 2001; 6(1):167–78.

[2] Bohay DR, Anderson JG. Stage IV posterior tibial tendon insufficiency: the tilted ankle. Foot Ankle Clin 2003;8:619–36.

[3] Boss AP, Hintermann B. Anatomical study if the medial ankle ligament complex. Foot Ankle Int 2002;23(9):547–53.

[4] Earl M, Wayne J, Brodick C. Contribution of the deltoid ligament to ankle joint contact characteristics: a cadaver study. Foot Ankle Int 1996;17(6):317–24.

[5] Friedman MA, Draganich LF, Toolan B, et al. The effects of adult acquired flatfoot deformity on tibiotalar joint contact characteristics. Foot Ankle Int 2001;22(3):241–6.

[6] Johnson KA, Strom DE. Tibialis posterior tendon dysfunction. Clin Orthop 1989;239: 196–206.

[7] Harper MC. Deltoid ligament: an anatomical evaluation of function. Foot Ankle Int 1987; 8(1):19–22.

[8] Mann RA. Flat foot in adults. In: Coughlin MJ, Mann RA, editors. Surgery of the foot and ankle, vol. 1. 7th edition. St Loius (MO): Mosby, Inc.; 1999. p. 733–67.

[9] Meehan RE, Brage M. Adult acquired flat foot deformity: clinical and radiographic examination. Foot Ankle Clin 2003;8:431–52.

[10] Papa JA, Myerson MS. Pantalar and tibiocalcaneal arthrodesis for post-traumatic osteoarthrosis of the ankle and hindfoot. J Bone Joint Surg Am 1992;81:1042–9.

[11] Manoli A II, Beals TC, Pomeroy GC. The role of osteotomies in the treatment of posterior tibial tendon disorders. Foot Ankle Clin 1997;2:309–17.

[12] Myerson M. Adult acquired flatfoot deformity: treatment of dysfunction of the posterior tibial tendon. J Bone Joint Surg Am 1996;78:780–92.

[13] Beals TC, Pomeroy GC, Manloli A. Posterior tibial tendon insufficiency: diagnosis and treatment. J Am Acad Orthop Surg 1999;7:112–8.

[14] Russotti GM, Johnson KA, Cass JR. Tibiotalocalcaneal arthrodesis for arthritis and deformity of the hind part of foot. J Bone Joint Surg Am 1988;70:1304–7.

[15] Chou RB, Mann RA, Yaszay S, et al. Tibiotalocalcaneal arthrodesis. Foot Ankle Int 2000; 21(10):804–8.

[16] Moore TJ, Prince R, Pochatko D, et al. Retrograde intramedullary nailing for ankle arthrodesis. Foot Ankle Int 1995;16(7):433–6.

[17] Resnick RB, Jahss MH, Choueka J, et al. Deltoid ligament forces after tibialis posterior tendon rupture: effects of triple arthrodesis and calcaneal displacement osteotomies. Foot Ankle Int 1995;16(1):14–20.

[18] Waugh TR, Wagner J, Stinchfield FE. An evaluation of pantalar arthrodesis. A follow-up study of one hundred and sixteen operations. J Bone Joint Surg Am 1965;47(7):1315–22.

[19] Barrett GR, Meyer LC, Bray EW 3rd, et al. Pantalar arthrodesis: a long-term follow-up. Foot Ankle 1981;1(5):279–83.

[20] Miehlke W, Gschwend N, Rippstein P, et al. Compression arthrodesis of the rheumatoid ankle and hindfoot. Clin Orthop Relat Res 1997;340:75–86.

[21] Acosta R, Ushiba J, Cracchiolo A 3rd. The results of a primary and staged pantalar arthrodesis and tibiotalocalcaneal arthrodesis in adult patients. Foot Ankle Int 2000; 21(3):182–94.

[22] Benthien RA, Myerson MS. Supramalleolar osteotomy for ankle deformity and arthritis. Foot Ankle Clin 2004;9:475–87.

[23] Lamm BM, Paley D. Deformity correction planning for hindfoot, ankle, and lower limb. Clin Podiatr Med Surg 2004;21:305–26.

[24] Silver RL, DeLaGarza J, Rang N. The myth of muscle balance: a study of relative strengths and excursions of normal muscles about the foot and ankle. J Bone Joint Surg Br 1985;67: 432–7.

[25] Statmatis ED, Myerson MS. Supramalleolar osteotomy: indications and technique. Foot Ankle Clin 2003;8:317–33.

[26] Neufeld SK, Myerson MS. Complications of surgical treatments for adult flatfoot deformities. Foot Ankle Clin 2001;6(1):179–91.

[27] Toolan BC, Sangeorzan BJ, Hansen ST. Complex reconstruction for the treatment of dorsolateral peritalar subluxation of the foot. J Bone Joint Surg 1999;81–A(11):1545–60.

[28] Mann RA. Posterior tibial tendon dysfunction, treatment by Flexor Digitorum Longus Transfer. Foot Ankle Clin 2001;6:77–87.

[29] Hansen ST. Osteotomy techniques, total ankle arthroplasty. In: Hansen ST, editor. Functional reconstruction of the foot and ankle. Lippincott Williams and Wilkins; 2000. p. 357–60, 430, 500–6.

[30] Easley ME, Vertullo CJ, Urban CW, et al. Total ankle arthroplasty. J Am Acad Orthop Surg 2002;10:157–67.

[31] Coughlin MJ. Arthritides. In: Coughlin MJ, Mann RA, editors. Surgery of the foot and ankle, vol. 1. 7th edition. St Loius (MO): Mosby, Inc.; 1999. p. 560–650.

ELSEVIER
SAUNDERS

Foot Ankle Clin N Am
12 (2007) 29–39

FOOT AND
ANKLE CLINICS

Distraction Arthroplasty

Kenneth R. Morse, MD[a],*, A. Samuel Flemister, MD[b],
Judith F. Baumhauer, MD[b],
Benedict F. DiGiovanni, MD[b]

[a]Department of Orthopaedics, University of Rochester Medical Center,
601 Elmwood Ave., Rochester, NY 14642, USA
[b]Division of Foot and Ankle Surgery, Department of Orthopaedics, University of Rochester
Medical Center, Box 665, 601 Elmwood Ave., Rochester, NY 14642, USA

Osteoarthritis is a progressive, degenerative disorder involving many different joints of the body, including the ankle. It is characterized by joint pain, tenderness, crepitus, inflammation, effusion, and limited range of motion. Radiographic findings include joint space narrowing, osteophyte formation, subchondral cysts, and subchondral sclerosis. The progressive nature of the disorder can lead to significant pain and long-term disability.

The treatment of osteoarthritis is aimed at decreasing pain, limiting disability, and slowing progression. Initial conservative measures consist of a combination of activity modification, physical therapy, medications, orthotic devices, and footwear modifications. When these measures fail and function cannot be maintained, surgical intervention is indicated.

Surgical options for arthritis of the ankle include joint-sparing procedures such as arthroscopy and tibial osteotomy and procedures that sacrifice the ankle joint such as fusion and ankle joint replacement. Arthroscopic debridement is indicated for patients who have mild to moderate osteoarthritis. This procedure is proposed to decrease pain, improve ankle motion, and postpone arthrodesis but its utility in patients who have advanced osteoarthritis is unpredictable [1]. Tibial osteotomies are designed to restore anatomic alignment and to improve biomechanical function of the ankle [2]. Stamatis and colleagues [3] reported on the treatment of 12 patients (13 feet) with supramalleolar osteotomy. The results showed an improvement in the average American Orthopaedic Foot and Ankle Society score from 53.8 to 87 points

None of the authors has any relationship with commercial companies or any direct financial interest in the subject matter.

* Corresponding author.

E-mail address: ken_morse@urmc.rochester.edu (K.R. Morse).

at a mean follow-up of 33.6 months [3]. Because the indications for tibial osteotomies are narrow and primarily involve patients who have asymmetric deformity and partial joint space narrowing, these procedures may not be appropriate for many patients who have ankle osteoarthritis [3,4].

For patients who have advanced degenerative changes, joint fusion and joint replacement are the mainstays of surgical therapy. Ankle arthrodesis has been shown to be effective in reducing pain but at the expense of joint motion and the subsequent overloading of adjacent joints. Coester and colleagues [5] reported moderate to severe subtalar arthritis in 21 of 23 patients at a mean of 22 years after ankle fusion. Similar findings were also seen in the other joints of the foot. Arthroplasty has also been shown to relieve pain secondary to arthritis; however, the lifespan of these implants is limited, with a reported 76% of patients exhibiting signs of radiolucency and 11% of patients undergoing revision surgery at a mean of 9 years [6]. Subsequent revision surgery requires significant bony resection, and the results are still unknown [7]. Therefore, these interventions may not be appropriate for the young patient who has severe ankle osteoarthritis and has failed conservative therapy.

In recent years, several researchers have studied the use of joint distraction arthroplasty, or arthrodiatasis, for the treatment of ankle arthritis [8,9]. With this technique, a distraction force is placed across the ankle joint using a small-wire external fixator. Weight bearing is allowed, which, through a hinge or the flexibility of the wires, creates intermittent fluid pressures within the joint while inhibiting mechanical loading of the joint [10].

Basic science

Although there is continued interest in the development of additional treatment options for ankle arthritis, the biology of osteoarthritic cartilage continues to be the focus of ongoing research. With the research conducted to date, it is clear that there are changes in the biochemical and biomechanical nature of the osteoarthritic articular cartilage surface. First, there is continuous deterioration of the articular cartilage secondary to progressive destruction of the collagen network and loss of cartilage molecules including proteoglycans. Because there are changes in the molecular structure of articular cartilage, there are also changes in its mechanical properties [11]. These property changes cause normal joint motion to further damage the vulnerable articular cartilage surface. In an attempt to repair this damage, chondrocytes dedifferentiate and begin to produce inappropriate matrix molecules such as catabolic cytokines and matrix proteases, which leads to further degradation of the cartilage.

Changes also occur below the articular surface, within the subchondral bone. Radiographically, the subchondral bone appears sclerotic, suggestive of increased bone density. On a microscopic level, several researchers have shown that there is a reduced mineral content and an increase in bony turnover [12]. Whether these subchondral changes are the result of alterations in the articular cartilage as previously described or whether they are the catalyst for such changes remains unclear.

History of distraction arthroplasty

Judet and Judet [13] reported one of the first studies using distraction arthroplasty. In their study, an articular cartilage lesion was created on the surface of canine tibiotarsal joints and a hinged external fixator was placed to provide distraction for 30 days. After 1 year, they found a reparative process that resembled that of "normal articular cartilage." The investigators also reported the successful use of distraction arthroplasty for the treatment of elbow, knee, and ankle joints with post-traumatic arthritis [13].

Subsequently, in 1994, Aldegheri and colleagues [14] described the use of distraction arthroplasty for the treatment of hip arthritis. In their study, 80 patients were treated with joint distraction by an axial external fixator. Their study showed "good" results in 71% of patients (42/59) under the age of 45 years. A "good" result was defined as (1) a resumption of normal activity with no pain or mild pain only after exercise, (2) greater than 90° of flexion and 20° of abduction, adduction, and internal and external rotation, and (3) independent ambulation for at least 30 minutes [14]. This report further emphasized the potential benefits of distraction arthroplasty in the young patient who has severe osteoarthritis. Following these reports, several researchers began to use the Ilizarov external fixator (Smith & Nephew, Memphis, Tennessee) to provide distraction for the treatment of ankle osteoarthritis [9,15].

Mechanism of action

The technique of joint distraction arthroplasty is based on the hypothesis that osteoarthritic cartilage has the potential to repair itself when the mechanical stress is removed from the articular surface [16]. Although the exact mechanism by which this reparative process occurs is unclear, several theories exist. The most popular theory is that the generation of intermittent fluid pressure while prohibiting mechanical loading has an effect on the healing capacity of the chondrocyte [10]. Several in vitro studies have subjected cultured osteoarthritic human chondrocytes to intermittent fluid pressures [8,17]. These studies have shown that the intermittent fluid pressure resulted in an increase in proteoglycan synthesis by the arthritic chondrocytes compared with the normal chondrocytes.

In 2000, van Valburg and colleagues [18] strengthened this theory with the use of a canine model. In this model, anterior cruciate ligament transection was used to create an osteoarthritic model in the canine knee. This model was then subjected to articulated and nonarticulated joint distraction. In the articulated joint distraction group, there was an increase in intermittent fluid pressures within the joint. When the articular cartilage from this group was analyzed (14 weeks after application of distraction), there were changes in proteoglycan metabolism that more closely resembled those of the normal contralateral knee. Although cartilage repair was not found in this study, the investigators believed that these metabolic changes would have been beneficial and might have led to cartilage repair if longer follow-up had been obtained [18].

Other researches have postulated that changes in the subchondral bone play a significant role in articular cartilage repair. After treatment with distraction arthroplasty, the subchondral bone appears to have decreased density, as suggested by radiographs. Marijnissen and colleagues [19] suggested that this decreased density leads to a greater portion of force absorbed at the subchondral surface, and therefore a reduction in the amount of force absorbed by the articular cartilage. It is difficult to determine, however, whether the decreased density leads to healing of the articular cartilage or whether the healthier cartilage, acted on by another mechanism, leads to stress shielding of the subchondral bone and, therefore, decreased density.

Other possible mechanisms of action that have been proposed include positive effects on nerve endings, decreased synovial inflammation, the formation of intra-articular fibrous tissue, stretching of the joint capsule, and decreased joint reactive forces [10].

Indications

Given the relatively recent introduction of distraction arthroplasty, the indications for the procedure are continuing to evolve. It has been suggested that the ideal candidate would be a young patient whose symptoms are refractory to conservative measures and who is unwilling to undergo arthrodesis [10]. Paley and Lamm [20] consider an ankle joint that is congruent, painful, mobile, and arthritic to be an appropriate joint for distraction arthroplasty. Contraindications include active infection, advanced coronal plane deformity, or significant loss of bone stock [10].

Technique

Several investigators have recommended that ankle arthroscopy or open ankle debridement be performed before the application of the distraction external fixator [10]. Standard arthroscopy can aid in the debridement of inflamed synovium, loose bodies, and areas of unstable cartilage or in the resection of tibiotalar osteophytes. In addition to debridement, areas of exposed bone can be treated with microfracture or drilling to increase blood flow and provide an enriched environment for healing. These steps aid in the removal of potential causes of persistent pain and improve dorsiflexion, which is imperative to the function of distraction arthroplasty. For the same reason, in patients who have equinus contracture, consideration should be given to performing Achilles tendon lengthening or gastrocnemius recession.

After these procedures are performed, attention is given to the application of the external fixator. The overall construct consists of a two-ring leg construct that is connected by threaded rods to a foot ring or foot plate. It is important that the foot ring be positioned at the midportion of the calcaneus and superior to the sole of the foot so as not to inhibit weight bearing.

The frame is assembled and held provisionally in place with Kirschner wires. Next, under fluoroscopic guidance, an extra-articular reference wire is placed just above and parallel to the ankle joint. With this reference wire in place and provisional fixation in place, the alignment of the joint and frame is assessed. The leg should be in the center of the proximal ring and the construct should be parallel to the anterior border of the tibia. Particular attention should be given to the position of the foot, which should be in neutral.

After adjustments in the frame are made and the position of the frame is satisfactory, final fixation is obtained. For each ring, there should be at least two points of fixation, which is usually accomplished with small wires ideally placed 90° from each other. Although not always possible, the angle between the two wires should be as large as possible to maximize stability of the frame and to prevent frame migration. When placing the wires, care should be taken to capture as little soft tissue as possible to decrease pain and minimize soft tissue irritation. The wires should then be tensioned to approximately 100 to 130 kg, or 1.3 kN (Fig. 1) [10,16].

With the leg rings secure, the foot plate or foot ring is stabilized. The foot is held in neutral position and two olive wires are passed from each corner of the foot ring through the calcaneus. These wires are approximately 45° from each other and should be tensioned simultaneously so as not to bend the foot plate or ring (Fig. 2). Another half ring may be placed at the end of the foot ring to aid in preventing bending of the foot ring. One or two wires can then be placed through the forefoot, capturing the metatarsals or cuneiforms (Fig. 3). Finally, some investigators recommend the placement of an additional wire or wires through the neck of the talus for help in preventing equinus position, providing uniform distraction, and preventing distraction through the subtalar joint. These talar neck wires can be connected to the apparatus with raised posts off of the foot plate or by using a double-stacked foot ring (Fig. 4) [10].

With the apparatus in place and secure, distraction is begun by using distraction nuts placed on the threaded rods that connect the leg rings to the foot ring (Figs. 5 and 6). Most investigators recommend distraction of the joint in 0.5-mm increments twice daily for 5 days [10]. It must be understood that 5 mm of distraction on the threaded rod will not be equivalent to 5 mm of distraction at the ankle joint, secondary to the flexibility within the wires and the apparatus. Therefore, radiographs should be checked and adjustments made as necessary.

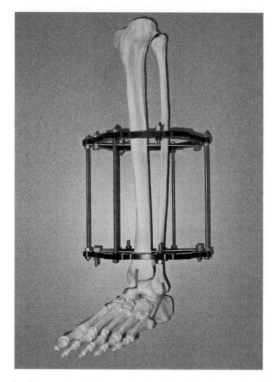

Fig. 1. Two-ring leg construct is secured using two wires through each of the rings.

Pin care is started two times daily with one-half strength hydrogen perox-ide and normal saline, and patients are followed weekly or biweekly until completion of treatment. Footwear is fashioned to accommodate the fixa-tor, and the patient is encouraged to progress to full weight bearing through the fixator. It is important to carefully monitor the pin sites because weight bearing will cause soft tissue irritation that can lead to pin tract infections if pin care is not adequate [10].

The distraction fixator is usually left in place for 3 months if tolerated by the patient. At 3 months, the fixator is removed and physical therapy is be-gun for range of motion and strengthening. Routine follow-up should be performed for several years after the procedure because clinical improve-ment has been shown to occur for months to years after the removal of the frame [9,19].

Results

Several series have been published illustrating the effects of joint distrac-tion on ankle osteoarthritis. In 1995, van Valburg and colleagues [21] reported a retrospective review of 11 patients who had post-traumatic ankle

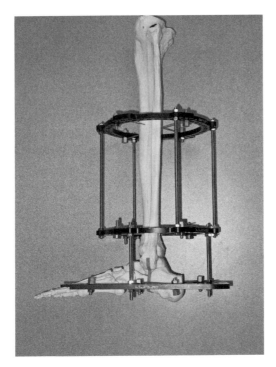

Fig. 2. Addition of a foot ring placed near the midportion of the calcaneus to allow weight bearing and placement of threaded rods to provide distraction.

arthritis treated with distraction arthroplasty. In each patient, the ankle joint was distracted by 5 mm using a small-wire frame for 3 months. Full weight bearing was allowed, and between 6 weeks and 12 weeks, ankle hinges were incorporated into the construct. At a mean follow-up of 20 months, all subjects reported improvement in pain, and in 3 of the 6 patients

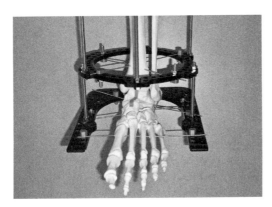

Fig. 3. Placement of a forefoot wire through one or more of the metatarsals to prevent equinus contracture.

MORSE et al

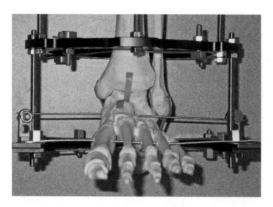

Fig. 4. Addition of posts and wire through the talar neck to prevent distraction through the subtalar joint.

for whom radiographs were available, an increase in joint space was observed. In addition to these findings, 3 patients underwent intra-articular pressure monitoring, which showed an increase in hydrostatic pressure during weight bearing [21].

In 1999, a follow-up multicenter, prospective study was reported that enrolled 17 patients who had a mean age of 39.6 years (range, 17–55 years), who exhibited radiographic evidence of severe ankle osteoarthritis, and who had pain and limited range of motion that was refractory to conservative measures [15]. In 13 of the 17 patients, ankle arthroscopy with debridement of intra-articular fibrosis and osteophytes was performed before the application of the small-wire, nonarticulating external fixator. Over, the course of several days, the ankle joint was distracted to at least 5 mm, weight bearing was allowed within 1 week, and distraction was maintained for 3 months. The patients were evaluated at 1 year and 2 years postoperatively by

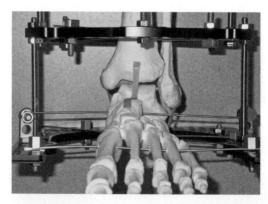

Fig. 5. Distraction of the ankle joint by turning the nuts on the threaded rods that connect the foot ring to the leg construct.

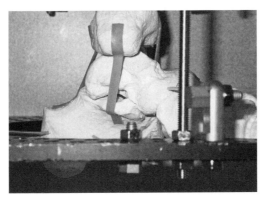

Fig. 6. Distraction of the ankle joint with minimal distraction through the subtalar joint secondary to the presence of a talar wire.

physical examination, radiographs, and subjective surveys. The investigators found that approximately two thirds of the patients noted significant improvement in functional ability and pain relief. These benefits were also present at the 2-year follow-up, and the patients showed a tendency to progressively improve as time passed. In 75% of patients, there was an increase in joint mobility; in 50% of patients, there was a significant increase in joint space measurement. Four of the patients noted no beneficial effects from the distraction arthroplasty and required fusion. These findings were consistent with previous retrospective findings and further supported distraction arthroplasty as a treatment option for severe ankle arthritis [15].

One of the largest studies to date was reported by Marijnissen and colleagues [9]. In this prospective study, 57 patients who had a mean age of 44 years (range, 18–65 years) and refractory ankle osteoarthritis were enrolled and followed for an average of 2.8 years. Again, a portion of the patients (35/57) underwent arthroscopic debridement before application of a nonarticulating external fixator. After removal of 11 subjects who were followed for less than 1 year, the remaining 46 patients were evaluated using the visual analog pain scale and a modification of a functional score described by van Valburg and colleagues [15]. The results showed a significant benefit in 33 of the remaining 46 patients (72%), with an average decrease in the pain score of 38% (statistically significant) and an increase in the function score of 69% ($P < .0001$) [9]. In addition, for those patients who had longer follow-up, the benefit appeared to increase with time. Radiographically, the investigators noted an average increase in joint space of 17% (n = 12 patients) ($P < .04$) and a decrease in subchondral sclerosis of 10% ($P < .003$). The remaining 28% of patients (n = 13 patients) developed recurrent pain after treatment with joint distraction and required fusion [9]. Within this study, the investigators conducted a separate randomized controlled trial in which 17 patients were randomized to receive joint distraction or arthroscopy with debridement. Significant differences between the two groups were found, with greater improvement in pain and function in the joint distraction group [9].

Marijnissen and colleagues [9] also reported on the potential risks and complications in their series of 57 patients. In their experience, no serious complications were encountered. Pin tract infections developed in 16 patients (28%) and were treated with oral antibiotics, and the forefoot wire broke in 8 patients (14%) [9].

The long-term benefits of distraction arthroplasty in the ankle were addressed by Ploegmakers and colleagues [22] in 2005. In their report, 22 patients who had a mean age of 37 years (range, 19–55 years) and ankle arthritis were treated by distraction arthroplasty and followed for an average of 10 years after surgery. Of these 22 patients, 6 (27%) were considered failures, with 5 patients going on to arthrodesis and 1 patient suffering from Sudeck's atrophy. Of the remaining 16 patients, significant improvements in all clinical parameters were observed [22].

Summary

Few joint-preserving surgical options exist for the patient who has ankle arthritis refractory to conservative measures. Therefore, continuous effort is afforded to the development of additional treatment options for such patients. Distraction arthroplasty has been proposed as one of these options for the patient in whom fusion or joint replacement is not appropriate.

Although the mechanism of action remains unknown, the reports of several researchers support the potential beneficial effects that can be obtained from joint distraction arthroplasty in the severely osteoarthritic ankle. Furthermore, the studies published to date suggest that these effects may not only persist for years but also improve as time progresses during the first several years after treatment.

Although additional laboratory studies are needed to understand the biochemical and biomechanical effects of distraction, additional prospective clinical studies are also needed to further understand its efficacy and appropriate patient population. The data thus far suggests that joint distraction arthroplasty may be a viable alternative treatment to arthrodesis and replacement for the young patient who has a congruent, painful, mobile, arthritic ankle joint.

References

[1] Tol JL, Verheyen CP, van Dijk CN. Arthroscopic treatment of anterior impingement in the ankle. J Bone Joint Surg Br 2001;83(1):9–13.
[2] Stamatis ED, Myerson MS. Supramalleolar osteotomy: indications and technique. Foot Ankle Clin 2003;8(2):317–33.

[3] Stamatis ED, Cooper PS, Myerson MS. Supramalleolar osteotomy for the treatment of distal tibial angular deformities and arthritis of the ankle joint. Foot Ankle Int 2003;24(10): 754–64.

[4] Takakura Y, Takaoka T, Tanaka Y, et al. Results of opening-wedge osteotomy for the treatment of a post-traumatic varus deformity of the ankle. J Bone Joint Surg Am 1998;80(2): 213–8.

[5] Coester LM, Saltzman CL, Leupold J, et al. Long-term results following ankle arthrodesis for post-traumatic arthritis. J Bone Joint Surg Am 2001;83-A(2):219–28.

[6] Knecht SI, Estin M, Callaghan JJ, et al. The agility total ankle arthroplasty. Seven to sixteen-year follow-up. J Bone Joint Surg Am 2004;86-A(6):1161–71.

[7] Kopp FJ, Patel MM, Deland JT, et al. Total ankle arthroplasty with the agility prosthesis: clinical and radiographic evaluation. Foot Ankle Int 2006;27(2):97–103.

[8] van Valburg AA, van Roy HL, Lafeber FP, et al. Beneficial effects of intermittent fluid pressure of low physiological magnitude on cartilage and inflammation in osteoarthritis. An in vitro study. J Rheumatol 1998;25(3):515–20.

[9] Marijnissen AC, Van Roermund PM, Van Melkebeek J, et al. Clinical benefit of joint distraction in the treatment of severe osteoarthritis of the ankle: proof of concept in an open prospective study and in a randomized controlled study. Arthritis Rheum 2002;46(11): 2893–902.

[10] Chiodo CP, McGarvey W. Joint distraction for the treatment of ankle osteoarthritis. Foot Ankle Clin 2004;9(3):541–53, ix.

[11] Buckwalter JA, Mankin HJ. Articular cartilage: tissue design and chondrocyte-matrix interactions. Instr Course Lect 1998;47:477–86.

[12] Li B, Aspden RM. Composition and mechanical properties of cancellous bone from the femoral head of patients with osteoporosis or osteoarthritis. J Bone Miner Res 1997;12(4): 641–51.

[13] Judet R, Judet T. The use of a hinge distraction apparatus after arthrolysis and arthroplasty. Rev Chir Orthop Reparatrice Appar Mot 1978;64(5):353–65 [in French].

[14] Aldegheri R, Trivella G, Saleh M. Articulated distraction of the hip. Conservative surgery for arthritis in young patients. Clin Orthop Relat Res 1994;301:94–101.

[15] van Valburg AA, van Roermund PM, Marijnissen AC, et al. Joint distraction in treatment of osteoarthritis: a two-year follow-up of the ankle. Osteoarthritis Cartilage 1999;7(5):474–9.

[16] van Roermund PM, Marijnissen AC, Lafeber FP. Joint distraction as an alternative for the treatment of osteoarthritis. Foot Ankle Clin 2002;7(3):515–27.

[17] Lafeber F, Veldhuijzen JP, Vanroy JL, et al. Intermittent hydrostatic compressive force stimulates exclusively the proteoglycan synthesis of osteoarthritic human cartilage. Br J Rheumatol 1992;31(7):437–42.

[18] van Valburg AA, van Roermund PM, Marijnissen AC, et al. Joint distraction in treatment of osteoarthritis (II): effects on cartilage in a canine model. Osteoarthritis Cartilage 2000;8(1): 1–8.

[19] Marijnissen AC, van Roermund PM, van Melkebeek J, et al. Clinical benefit of joint distraction in the treatment of ankle osteoarthritis. Foot Ankle Clin 2003;8(2):335–46.

[20] Paley D, Lamm BM. Ankle joint distraction. Foot Ankle Clin 2005;10(4):685–98, ix.

[21] van Valburg AA, van Roermund PM, Lammens J, et al. Can Ilizarov joint distraction delay the need for an arthrodesis of the ankle? A preliminary report. J Bone Joint Surg Br 1995; 77(5):720–5.

[22] Ploegmakers JJ, van Roermund PM, van Melkebeek J, et al. Prolonged clinical benefit from joint distraction in the treatment of ankle osteoarthritis. Osteoarthritis Cartilage 2005;13(7): 582–8.

ELSEVIER
SAUNDERS

Foot Ankle Clin N Am
12 (2007) 41–55

Classification and Treatment of Severe Ankle Articular Segment Deficits: Osteochondral Allograft Reconstruction

Todd A. Irwin, MD[1], Joseph X. Kou, MD[1],
Paul T. Fortin, MD*

Department of Orthopaedic Surgery, William Beaumont Hospital, 3535 W Thirteen Mile Road, Suite 744, Royal Oak, MI 48073, USA

Articular injuries involving the ankle may lead to arthritis involving the tibial plafond, the talar dome, or both. Traumatic events account for 70% of all cases of ankle arthritis [1]. Treatment of these injuries and the resultant arthritis continues to be a challenging problem as they often occur in younger, more active patients. For severe degenerative or posttraumatic arthritis, ankle arthrodesis provides satisfactory pain relief and continues to be the gold standard. Arthrodesis leads to functional limitations, however, and can lead to progressive arthritis of the subtalar, talonavicular, naviculocuneiform, calcaneocuboid, and tarsometatarsal joints [2,3]. Total ankle arthroplasty is an increasingly viable option with the advent of newer prostheses and evolving surgeon experience. Performing total ankle arthroplasty in younger, more active patients is relatively contraindicated, however. In a study of 306 total ankle arthroplasties, patients less than 54 years of age were found to have a 1.45 times greater risk for reoperation and a 2.65 times greater risk for failure than patients older than 54 years [4].

Osteochondral allograft transplantation provides an alternative treatment option in this difficult patient population. Replacing damaged articular cartilage with fresh osteochondral allograft has been performed with variable success for several decades. Although many joints have been studied, grafts involving the femoral condyle or the tibial plateau are the best documented and have the longest follow-up [5]. The success of this

---

* Corresponding author.
[1] Present addresses: 32810 Bingham Lane, Bingham Farms, MI 48025 (Todd A. Irwin); 6267 Quaker Hill Drive, West Bloomfield, MI 48322 (Joseph X. Kou).
E-mail address: pfortin@comcast.net (P.T. Fortin).

treatment option has led to the increased use of osteochondral allografts to treat focal and severe ankle deficits. The aim of this article is to provide an overview for treating severe articular loss of the ankle with osteochondral allografts, including specifics regarding the use of allografts, the surgical options, and both the clinical outcomes and graft viability.

Donor osteochondral allografts

Patients who have significant tibial plafond or talar dome articular loss that is not amenable to debridement, osteochondral autografts, or autologous chondrocyte implantation because of the size of the deficit and who have otherwise failed conservative treatment are potential candidates for osteochondral allograft transplantation. Once this treatment option has been established, decisions regarding the type of allograft must be made. Historically, osteochondral allografts intended for implantation were frozen using cryopreservation agents, such as glycerol or dimethyl sulfoxide [6]. Bulk frozen allografts continue to be used in the reconstructive phase of tumor resection [7]. It has been shown, however, that there is complete or near-complete loss of chondrocyte viability in these grafts after freezing, with viable tissue being limited to the superficial layer of the cartilage matrix [8]. As an alternative to cryopreservation, programs using fresh osteochondral allografts implanted shortly after harvest were started [5,9].

Transplantation of fresh osteochondral allografts has provided good clinical results for several decades, most commonly for femoral condyle or tibial plateau defects. In the initial procedures tissue was transplanted within 5 days of donor death [10]. Because of more stringent disease transmission testing and regulations and the availability of allografts through commercial tissue bank distributors, the time between graft procurement and implantation has increased. This change has led to questions concerning chondrocyte viability in stored, fresh osteochondral allografts relative to length of storage and storage environment.

Donor chondrocyte viability

Fresh allografts initially were stored in lactated Ringer solution at 4°C. It was shown that after 7 days of storage in lactated Ringer solution chondrocyte viability and metabolic activity were significantly decreased. Fresh osteochondral allografts were then stored in a serum-free modified culture medium, which led to significant improvement in chondrocyte viability at 14 days (90.5% ± 6.3%) and metabolic activity compared with fresh grafts stored in lactated Ringer solution (80% ± 17% chondrocyte viability) [10]. Another study looked at the quality of human articular cartilage after storage in culture medium at 4°C for 1, 7, 14, and 28 days. This study revealed chondrocyte viability decreases only 1.7% after 14 days of storage in culture medium compared with a 28.5% decrease after 28 days of storage.

Meanwhile, chondrocyte metabolic activity is relatively preserved after 7 days of storage, and biomechanical properties of the cartilage remained unchanged after 28 days [11]. A third study showed $82.5\% \pm 5\%$ chondrocyte viability at a mean of 20.3 ± 2.9 days of storage in serum-free media [12].

Although this research has led to improved conditions of storage for fresh osteochondral allografts, there is currently no universal method to measure the viability of stored cartilage. Factors used to assess cartilage viability include measuring chondrocyte viability with various stains or ultrastructural analysis with electron microscopy; measuring biochemical properties, such as proteoglycan synthesis and glycosaminoglycan content; and analyzing biomechanical properties, such as indentation stiffness [10–13]. More recent evidence suggests certain techniques may be overestimating chondrocyte viability in osteoarticular allografts [13]. As it is believed that viable chondrocytes are integral to the long-term integrity of transplanted osteochondral allografts, orthopaedic surgeons should be aware of the conditions in which the fresh osteochondral allografts they are implanting have been stored.

Although there is some variability among tissue banks, most commercially available osteochondral allografts undergo a 21-day screening process after graft procurement. Typically the grafts are available for implantation an average of 3 days after the screening process is complete [12]. The above research demonstrates the time-dependent nature of chondrocyte viability; timely implantation of the graft as soon as it becomes available is important.

Treatment options for massive osteochondral deficits

Patients who have posttraumatic arthritis of the ankle may be candidates for osteochondral allograft transplantation. Injury patterns include various-sized osteochondral deficits in the talus or the tibia, degenerative changes isolated to the talar dome or tibial plafond, and diffuse tibiotalar arthrosis. Nonoperative treatment includes the use of anti-inflammatories, bracing, and a course of protected weight bearing.

Surgical management of osteochondral deficits includes debridement, internal fixation of the fragment, excision and curettage with or without drilling, cancellous bone grafting, and osteochondral transplantation [14]. Resurfacing of these deficits with osteochondral allograft is a biologic alternative that functions to fill in the deficit and provide an articulating surface. The goal is to prevent an arthritic ankle by preventing excess load bearing on the remainder of the articular surface. Treatment alternatives for smaller deficits have included osteoarticular transfer and autologous chondrocyte implantation [14]. Larger defects, those with significant bone loss, and defects located where duplication of the anatomy is difficult to reconstruct with autograft (such as shoulder defects of the talus) may be more amenable to osteochondral allograft. The use of a single graft instead of multiple grafts minimizes fibrocartilage ingrowth.

The surgical technique of reconstructing articular deficits of the ankle requires adequate exposure. Unlike the knee, access to the area of articular loss in the ankle is often difficult. This difficulty may necessitate osteotomy to gain exposure. The extent of resection required should be determined with preoperative MRI and CT imaging studies.

Classification of articular segment deficit

Focal osteochondral defects or lesions have been classified by Berndt and Harty. There is, however, no current classification system that describes large articular segment deficits of the tibiotalar joint. Factors that are important in the classification of this condition are location and extent of the articular segment deficit and vascularity of the underlying bone. Box 1 describes the classification system that we find helpful in planning operative treatment. We consider Grade I ankles to have segmental deficits that are isolated to either the talus or tibia. Grade II ankles have more diffuse articular deficits occurring in the talar dome (Fig. 1A, B), and Grade III ankles have diffuse deficits isolated to the articular surface of the tibial plafond. Diffuse articular deficits involving both the talar dome and tibial plafond are considered Grade IV ankles. We further classified each grade into Subtype A and B. Subtype A indicates there is no evidence of avascular necrosis deep to the articular deficit, whereas subtype B indicates the presence of avascular necrosis deep to the degenerative cartilage that would remain after resection of the articular segment deficit. A posttraumatic ankle with a B modifier would not be a good candidate for osteochondral allograft

---

Box 1. Articular segment deficit classification

Grade I: Segmental articular deficit isolated to either a portion of the tibia or talus

Grade II: Diffuse articular deficit or degenerative change isolated to the talus

Grade III: Diffuse articular deficit or degenerative change isolated to the tibia

Grade IV: Diffuse articular deficits apparent on both the tibia and the talus

Subtype A: No signs of avascular necrosis deep to the articular segment deficit

Subtype B: Evidence of avascular necrosis deep to the articular segment deficit

Subtypes A and B can be applied to Grades I–IV

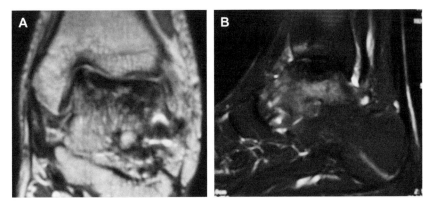

Fig. 1. (*A*, *B*) Grade IIA articular segment deficit in a patient who had a previous subtalar arthrodesis following talar trauma. MRI shows vascularized talus deep to the articular segment that will be resected.

because of poor potential for healing through creeping substitution. A Grade IA ankle joint would be amenable to a partial talus allograft. Grade IIA and IIIA could benefit from a hemiarthroplasty osteochondral allograft, and Grade IVA would be amenable to a bipolar osteochondral allograft.

Segmental articular deficits

Partial osteochondral defects of both the distal tibia and talar dome can be reconstructed with allografts as demonstrated by Chapman and Mann [15] and Gross and colleagues [16]. Gross and colleagues [16] recommended osteochondral allografting in an area of fragmentation and collapse involving a cartilage deficit of at least 1 cm in diameter and 5 mm in depth where the fragment cannot be reattached. Partial articular deficits of the talus are commonly identified on either the medial or lateral side (Fig. 2). Lateral side deficits can be exposed through an incision anterior to the fibula. If the deficit is posterolateral, consideration of a Gatellier approach or an osteotomy of the anterolateral tibia may be needed for adequate exposure. The deficit is resected using free-hand technique with a thin-blade oscillating saw to form a base and edge that will be matched with the allograft. Once the allograft is shaped to fit the defect, stabilization with counter-sunk mini-fragment screws are used [17].

Unipolar diffuse articular deficits

Large articular deficits and diffuse involvement, such as those seen in avascular necrosis of the talus that has failed nonoperative treatment, can also be managed with a talar dome allograft hemiarthroplasty. Preoperative CT of the ankle can aide in evaluating the extent of arthrosis (Fig. 3A–D). Additionally, arthroscopy of the ankle before the reconstruction may be

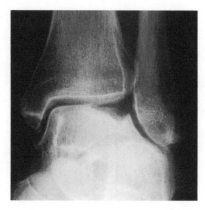

Fig. 2. Grade IA segmental talar defect.

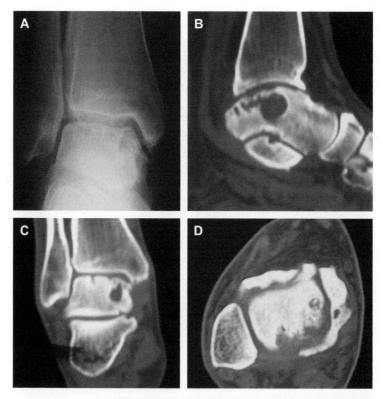

Fig. 3. (A–D) Radiographs and CT images of Grade IIA articular segment deficit. (E) Ankle joint distraction and resection of the talar dome. (F) Sizing of the talar dome. (G) Free-hand resection of the donor talar dome. (H) Hemiarthroplasty allograft in place. (I, J) Postoperative radiographs after fixation.

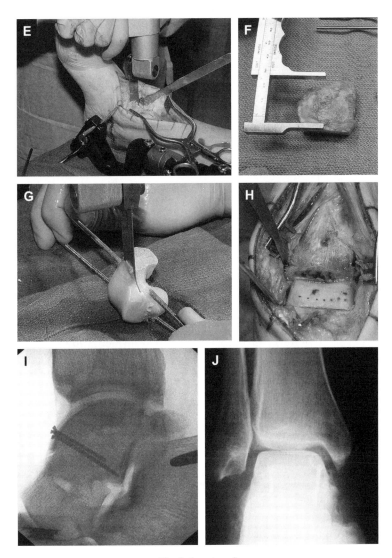

Fig. 3 (*continued*)

helpful to assess involvement of the tibial plafond. Hemiarthroplasty with talar dome allograft is a viable option only if the degenerative changes are isolated to the talus and the distal tibial plafond is intact. Any mechanical axis malalignment or ankle instability must be corrected either simultaneously or before allograft implantation. Because of the relative rigidity of the distal tibial plafond compared with the talar dome, isolated distal tibial lesions are less common. Unipolar distal tibial allograft is also an option for treatment, however [18].

The surgical technique for talar dome allograft involves the use of an external fixator. At our institution, we use an EBI (Biomet, Warsaw, IN) external fixator with two pins in the tibia, one in the talar neck and one in the calcaneal tuberosity. The external fixator is used to distract the ankle joint. The ankle is then approached anteriorly between the tibialis anterior and extensor hallucis longus. The neurovascular bundle is protected and retracted laterally and care is taken to leave the tendon sheath of the tibialis anterior intact. An oscillating saw is used to resect the talar dome using a cut that is parallel to the joint starting at the interface of the anterior cartilage and talar neck (Fig. 3E). The donor-matched allograft talus is then cut in the same fashion, but is cut a few millimeters thicker to account for loss of height (Fig. 3F, G). The talar dome allograft is then press-fit into the ankle and should be stable after the distraction is released. Internal fixation is used with two mini-fragment screws at the anterior edge of the graft directed posteroinferiorly into the calcaneus (Fig. 3H–J).

Bipolar diffuse articular deficits

When ankle degeneration involves both the tibial plafond and talar dome, fresh tibiotalar osteochondral allograft transplantation can provide an alternative to ankle fusion or total ankle prosthetic arthroplasty [9,18,19]. The advantages of bipolar allograft transplantation include preservation of some tibiotalar motion and maintenance of bone stock, leaving ankle arthrodesis or total ankle prosthetic arthroplasty as a viable salvage procedure if needed (Fig. 4A, B).

The surgical technique of bipolar allografting is similar to talar dome allograft and was described by Kim and colleagues [19] and Tontz and colleagues [9]. An external fixator is used for joint distraction, and the ankle is approached anteriorly. The dome of the talus can be resected free hand with the oscillating saw as described above. The distal tibial plafond cuts are made with the Agility (Depuy, Warsaw IN) total ankle cutting guide. The guide should be placed so that a depth of approximately 10 mm is resected from the tibial plafond and approximately 3 to 4 mm from the articular portion of the medial malleolus is resected. The cutting line for the fibula is not used and the articular portion of the fibula is left intact. The cutting jig is also used for harvesting the donor graft, but it should be one size larger than the recipient jig. The talar dome donor is harvested as described above. Once again, the allograft is press-fit on both sides of the ankle joint and the distractor is released. The tibial graft is stabilized with internal fixation using mini-fragment screws starting at the anterior portion of the graft and directed posterosuperiorly into the host tibia. The talar graft is stabilized as described above (Fig. 4C–F).

Postoperative management of osteochondral allografts consist of a postoperative bulky splint transitioned to a short leg bivalved cast on postoperative day 2. Patients are placed in a boot at 4 weeks, kept non–weight bearing for 3 months and then progressed to full weight bearing afterwards.

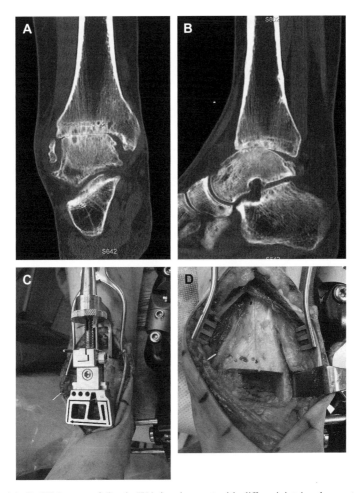

Fig. 4. (*A, B*) CT images of Grade IVA involvement with diffuse joint involvement. (*C, D*) Resection of the tibiotalar joint. (*E, F*) Postoperative radiographs after graft placement.

Complications

As techniques in transplanting osteochondral allografts have evolved, several complications have been encountered. Matching the size of the donor allograft with the host talus or tibia is important and thus measurements should be verified with both radiographs and CT scans of the host ankle. Despite this process, graft–host mismatch can occur, which can lead to graft resorption or graft impingement (Fig. 5A, B). Graft fragmentation and graft collapse have also been seen [9,16,20], which may require revision allografting or arthrodesis if symptomatic. As bone resection using free-hand technique introduces an element of operator-dependent error, meticulous technique is important in creating a flush graft–host interface.

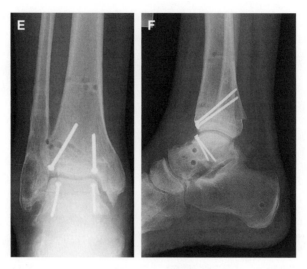

Fig. 4 (*continued*)

Nonunion can occur at the graft–host interface, however, and one case reported by Kim and colleagues [19] resulted in malunion of the talar allograft resulting in talar subluxation secondary to poor fit of the talus. One criticism of bipolar allografting is that the talofibular joint is not addressed, which can result in persistent lateral gutter pain that may require

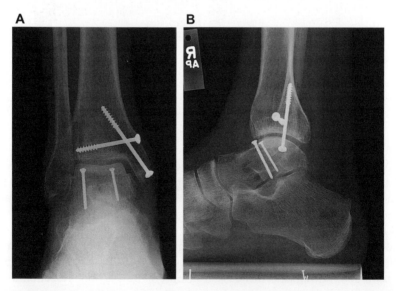

Fig. 5. (*A, B*) Radiographs of a talar dome hemiarthroplasty showing sizing mismatch of the graft on the AP view.

debridement. Intraoperative fractures of both the medial and lateral malleoli have also been seen, usually occurring during the tibial osteotomy [9,18,19]. Failed grafts have shown varying degrees of secondary osteoarthritic changes usually associated with fragmentation or resorption [16,18]. Not uncommonly, reactive osteophytes form at the anterior aspect of the tibiotalar joint (Fig. 6A–D). Finally, as with any surgical procedure, infection is a risk, although no deep infections have been reported to date in ankle allograft transplantation.

Clinical results

Functional outcomes

Most clinical outcomes reported in the literature are based on implantation of fresh osteochondral allografts in the knee [5,21–23]. A few studies have reported their results after implanting fresh osteochondral allografts into the ankle joint, both for large talar defects and for tibiotalar ankle arthropathy [9,15–20].

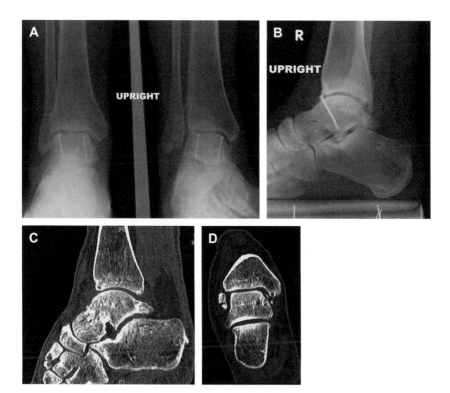

Fig. 6. (A–D) Talar dome hemiarthroplasty 3 years after implantation showing incorporation of the graft without collapse but reactive osteophyte formation of the anterior ankle joint.

In the study by Gross and colleagues [16], nine patients were treated with fresh partial talar allografts shaped to replace large talar dome lesions. After an average 12-year follow-up, six of the nine allografts remained in situ and all six patients had functional range of motion, no limitations to minor limitations with activity, and were satisfied with the surgery. The other three ankles had radiographic and intraoperative evidence of fragmentation, greater than 50% resorption with degenerative changes, and required ankle arthrodesis as a salvage procedure.

Raikin [20] reported on six cases of massive osteochondral talar defects treated with partial talar allografts fashioned into an even-edged rectangular shape. The size criteria used was volume greater than 3 cm^3, with four fresh frozen allografts and two fresh allografts implanted. After an average follow-up of 23 months, 5 of 6 allografts were intact with one patient undergoing ankle arthrodesis secondary to persistent pain. American Orthopaedic Foot and Ankle Society (AOFAS) ankle/hindfoot score improved an average of 44 points, with all patients being satisfied with the results.

Hemiarthroplasty may be used to restore articular congruity of the ankle joint in cases of talar dome collapse before significant involvement of the tibial plafond. There have not been any published series of talar dome hemiarthroplasty alone. This procedure obviously has the advantage of less bone resection than a bipolar graft and potentially fewer complications. We have performed talar dome hemiarthroplasty using fresh osteochondral allograft in five patients who had isolated severe talar dome deficits. Three of five patients had limited chondral involvement of the tibia. All had focal avascular necrosis that dictated the area of graft resection. Our preliminary results are encouraging; all patients have had improvement in pain and function, although long-term follow-up is lacking.

Meehan and colleagues [18] described their experience in treating tibiotalar joint arthritis using fresh osteochondral allografts in 11 patients (9 bipolar transplants, 1 tibial unipolar transplant, and 1 talar unipolar transplant) at an average follow-up of 33 months. Six of the 11 ankles were considered successful with average AOFAS score improving from 55 to 73. Of the 5 patients who had failed allografts, 3 had successful revision bipolar allografts and 1 had successful conversion to a total ankle arthroplasty. The same group earlier reported long-term results (148 months) on 7 patients undergoing bipolar osteochondral shell allografts with a failure rate of 42%. This finding led to the revised surgical technique mentioned earlier using the cutting jigs from the Agility ankle arthroplasty system (Depuy, Warsaw, IN) [9]. This modified technique led to improved graft fit and better results [19].

Chondrocyte viability after clinical implantation

Although the clinical success of osteochondral allograft transplantation has been established, there is little information available regarding the survival of the transplanted articular cartilage. In animal models, short-term analysis of chondrocytes harvested after fresh osteochondral allograft transplantation revealed preservation of biomechanical and biochemical properties. In addition, histologic evaluation revealed normal cartilage structure [24,25]. Long-term data is needed to establish this technique as a viable treatment option in young adults. Czitrom and colleagues [26] biopsied articular cartilage in four patients who received fresh osteochondral allografts secondary to trauma in the knee or elbow. They reported 69% to 99% chondrocyte viability between 12 and 41 months postoperatively, and 37% chondrocyte viability at 6 years. The longest reported follow-up of viable chondrocytes after fresh osteochondral allograft transplantation is 17 years following resection of a distal femoral giant cell tumor [27]. Another study reported 12 of 18 patients had evidence of viable hyaline cartilage in allografts excised at a mean 35 months postoperatively. This study also showed that five grafts had complete replacement of allograft bone with host bone by creeping substitution after 25 to 92 months [28]. Although larger studies are needed to prove the long-term viability of transplanted chondrocytes, it is evident that transplantation of fresh osteochondral allografts can preserve chondrocyte properties in appropriate conditions.

Immunogenicity

The ability to transplant osteochondral allografts without host rejection is based on the theory that articular cartilage is an immunologically privileged tissue. Langer and colleagues [29–31] have shown that articular chondrocytes themselves are immunogenic; however, they are protected from host cytotoxic antibodies when surrounded by intact cartilage matrix. The marrow elements of osteochondral allografts are not protected and thus produce an immune response [31]. Although this immune response has not proved to be of clinical significance, recent evidence suggests the host immune response may play a more significant role than originally believed. Phipatanakul and colleagues [32] showed that 8 of 14 fresh osteochondral allograft recipients produced immune reactivity against cartilage-specific protein (compared with 2 of 14 controls), indicating an immunologic response to the cartilage component of the osteochondral allograft. In the study on bipolar ankle allografts mentioned previously [18], 10 of 11 patients tested positive for serum HLA cytotoxic antibody six months postoperatively. The most successful radiographic and clinical result in their series was reported in a patient on immunosuppressant medication secondary to a previous kidney transplant. Finally, after allograft transplantation in the dog radius, Stevenson and colleagues [33] showed that dogs that received a canine leukocyte antigen-matched fresh allograft had the most successful histologic and biochemical results compared with antigen-mismatched and frozen allograft controls. Although current literature does not support the requirement of immunosuppressant medication in patients who receive fresh osteochondral allografts, further studies are needed to prove whether some form of immune suppression can increase the survival of fresh osteochondral allografts.

Summary

Severe ankle degeneration can be a devastating problem for young adults. Although ankle fusion continues to be the gold standard, inherent long-term problems are related to this treatment option. Further advances in total ankle prosthetic arthroplasty are needed before this treatment option can be considered suitable in a younger population. The use of fresh osteochondral allograft transplantation can provide an alternative treatment option without precluding future salvage procedures. Future studies may further define the role immunosuppression can play in improving fresh osteochondral allograft viability.

References

[1] Saltzman CL, Salamon ML, Blanchard M, et al. Epidemiology of ankle arthritis: report of a consecutive series of 639 patients from a tertiary orthopaedic center. Iowa Orthop J 2005; 25:44–6.

[2] Coester LM, Saltzman CL, Leupold J, et al. Long-term results following ankle arthrodesis for post-traumatic arthritis. J Bone Joint Surg Am 2001;83(2):219–28.

[3] Thomas R, Daniels TR, Parker K. Gait analysis and functional outcomes following ankle arthrodesis for isolated ankle arthritis. J Bone Joint Surg Am 2006;88(3):526–35.

[4] Spirit AA, Assal M, Hansen ST. Complications and failure after total ankle arthroplasty. J Bone Joint Surg Am 2004;86(6):1172–8.

[5] Gross AE, Shasha N, Aubin P. Long-term followup of the use of fresh osteochondral allografts for posttraumatic knee defects. Clin Orthop Relat Res 2005;435:79–87.

[6] Tomford WW, Fredericks GR, Mankin HJ. Studies on cryopreservation of articular cartilage chondrocytes. J Bone Joint Surg Am 1984;66(2):253–9.

[7] Mankin HJ, Gebhardt MC, Tomford WW. The use of frozen cadaveric allograft in the management of patients with bone tumors of the extremities. Orthop Clin North Am 1987;18: 275–89.

[8] Ohlendorf C, Tomford WW, Mankin HJ. Chondrocyte survival in cryopreserved osteochondral articular cartilage. J Orthop Res 1996;14(3):413–6.

[9] Tontz WL, Bugbee WD, Brage ME. Use of allografts in the management of ankle arthritis. Foot Ankle Clin 2003;8:361–73.

[10] Ball ST, Amiel D, Williams SK, et al. The effects of storage on fresh human osteochondral allografts. Clin Orthop Relat Res 2004;418:246–52.

[11] Williams SK, Amiel D, Ball ST, et al. Prolonged storage effects on the articular cartilage of fresh human osteochondral allografts. J Bone Joint Surg Am 2003;85(11): 2111–20.

[12] Allen RT, Robertson CM, Pennock AT, et al. Analysis of stored osteochondral allografts at the time of surgical implantation. Am J Sports Med 2005;33:1479–84.

[13] Amendola A, Martin J, Lightfoot A. Chondrocyte viability in osteoarticular allografts: are we overestimating chondrocyte viability? Presented at the American Orthopaedic Society for Sports Medicine 2006 Annual Meeting. Hershey (PA), June 29–July 2, 2006.

[14] Schafer DB. Cartilage repair of the talus. Foot Ankle Clin 2003;8:739–49.

[15] Chapman CB, Mann JA. Distal tibial osteochondral lesion treated with osteochondral allografting: a case report. Foot Ankle Int 2005;26(11):997–1000.

[16] Gross AE, Agnidis Z, Hutchison CR. Osteochondral defects of the talus treated with fresh osteochondral allograft transplantation. Foot Ankle Int 2001;22(5):385–91.

[17] Tasto JP, Ostrander R, Bugbee W, et al. The diagnosis and management of osteochondral lesions of the talus: osteochondral allograft update. Arthroscopy 2003;19(10 Suppl 1): 138–41.

[18] Meehan R, McFarlin S, Bugbee W, et al. Fresh ankle osteochondral allograft transplantation for tibiotalar joint arthritis. Foot Ankle Int 2005;26(10):793–802.

[19] Kim CW, Jamali A, Tontz W, et al. Treatment of post-traumatic ankle arthrosis with bipolar tibiotalar osteochondral shell allografts. Foot Ankle Int 2002;23(12):1091–102.

[20] Raikin SM. Stage VI: massive osteochondral defects of the talus. Foot Ankle Clin 2004;9: 737–44.

[21] Convery FR, Meyers MH, Akeson WH. Fresh osteochondral allografting of the femoral condyle. Clin Orthop Relat Res 1991;273:139–45.

[22] Ghazavi MT, Pritzker KP, Davis AM, et al. Fresh osteochondral allografts for post-traumatic osteochondral defects of the knee. J Bone Joint Surg Br 1997;79(6):1008–13.

[23] Jamali AA, Emmerson BC, Chung C, et al. Fresh osteochondral allografts: results in the patellofemoral joint. Clin Orthop Relat Res 2005;437:176–85.

[24] Oates KM, Chen AC, Young EP, et al. Effect of tissue culture storage on the in vivo survival of canine osteochondral allografts. J Orthop Res 1995;13(4):562–9.

[25] Glenn RE, McCarty EC, Potter HG, et al. Comparison of fresh osteochondral autografts and allografts: a canine model. Am J Sports Med 2006;10(10):1–10.

[26] Czitrom AA, Keating S, Gross AE. The viability of articular cartilage in fresh osteochondral allografts after clinical transplantation. J Bone Joint Surg Am 1990;72(4):574–81.

[27] McGoveran BM, Prtizker KPH, Shasha N, et al. Long-term chondrocyte viability in a fresh osteochondral allograft. J Knee Surg 2002;15(2):97–100.

[28] Oakeshott RD, Farine I, Pritzker KPH, et al. A clinical and histologic analysis of failed fresh osteochondral allografts. Clin Orthop Relat Res 1988;233:283–94.

[29] Langer F, Gross AE. Immunogenicity of allograft articular cartilage. J Bone Joint Surg Am 1974;56(2):297–304.

[30] Langer F, Czitrom A, Pritzker KP, et al. The immunogenicity of fresh and frozen allogeneic bone. J Bone Joint Surg Am 1975;57(2):216–20.

[31] Langer F, Gross AE, West M, et al. The immunogenicity of allograft knee joint transplants. Clin Orthop Relat Res 1978;132:155–62.

[32] Phipatanakul WP, VandeVord PJ, Teitge RA, et al. Immune response in patients receiving fresh osteochondral allografts. Am J Orthop 2004;33(7):345–8.

[33] Stevenson S, Dannucci GA, Sharkey NA, et al. The fate of articular cartilage after transplantation of fresh and cryopreserved tissue-antigen-matched and mismatched osteochondral allografts in dogs. J Bone Joint Surg Am 1989;71(9):1297–307.

ELSEVIER
SAUNDERS

Foot Ankle Clin N Am
12 (2007) 57–73

FOOT AND
ANKLE CLINICS

Combined Subtalar and Ankle Arthritis

Lucille B. Andersen, MD*, Michael P. Stauff, MD, Paul J. Juliano, MD

Penn State Milton S. Hershey Medical Center, Penn State College of Medicine, Orthopaedics and Rehabilitation, H089, 500 University Drive, P.O. Box 850, Hershey, PA 17033-0850, USA

Combined subtalar and ankle arthritis is a difficult entity to treat. The goals of treatment are to eliminate pain and correct deformity while creating a limb that can be used to ambulate in an energy-efficient manner. There are many different ways to attain these goals based on the cause of the arthritis, previous interventions, and comorbid conditions.

Cause

Concurrent subtalar and ankle arthritis can manifest in many ways. Historically, talus fractures have resulted in this pattern of arthritis since Fabricius Hildanus [1] described the fracture dislocation in 1608. Bingold [2] also noted the association between severe fractures of the talus and degenerative pantalar arthritis. Similarly, others have noted that posttraumatic arthritis can follow severe pilon or talus fractures [3–5]. Trauma is not the only way in which combined subtalar and ankle arthritis can arise. Isolated arthritis of the ankle or subtalar joint treated with fusion can lead to degenerative changes of the contiguous joint [6]. Failed total ankle arthroplasty with previous subtalar fusion is another permutation that can result in combined arthritis. Neuropathy has long been a known cause of pantalar arthritis. Neuropathic pantalar arthritis in the past was largely a sequelae of leprosy and syphilis [7]; however, the incidence of diabetes mellitus and neuropathy has far surpassed these conditions. In one series, Papa and colleagues [8] attempted salvage on 29 patients who had neuropathic arthropathy of the foot and ankle. Other causes of combined subtalar and ankle arthritis include rheumatoid arthritis, crystalline arthropathies,

---

* Corresponding author.
E-mail address: landersen@hmc.psu.edu (L.B. Andersen).

polio, and congenital deformities, such as talipes equinovarus [9,10]. Recently, it has been noted that soft tissue disorders, such as posterior tibial tendon insufficiency, can lead to combined ankle and subtalar degeneration (Figs. 1 and 2) [11]. Each of these conditions can lead to progressive arthropathy in the ankle and subtalar joint resulting in disabling pain, worsening deformity, and restricted ambulation.

Biomechanics

The ankle and subtalar joints have vital roles in locomotion. The ankle joint should have 20° of dorsiflexion (DF) and 40° of plantar flexion (PF) [12]. Subtalar motion has been difficult to define, with a range of 20° to 60° reported and a 2:1 ratio of inversion to eversion [13,14]. Numerous studies have evaluated the biomechanical relationship between the ankle, subtalar joint, and other hindfoot joints [14–18]. Mann [17] and Isman and Inman [15] found that subtalar eversion and tibial-talar internal rotation help dissipate the ground reaction force from an axial to a rotational vector at heel strike. In this way, each joint absorbs less stress.

Nonoperative treatment

Treatment of combined ankle and subtalar arthritis is varied depending on the severity of disease, the individual activity, pain, and comorbidities.

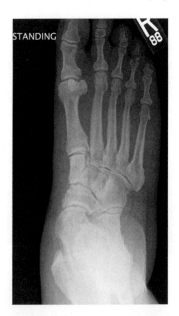

Fig. 1. AP (anteroposterior) radiograph of foot with significant posterior tibialis tendon dysfunction and uncovering of talus.

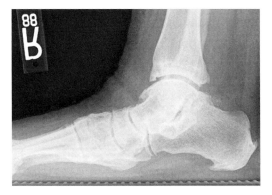

Fig. 2. Lateral radiograph of foot from Fig. 1 with associated subtalar and ankle degeneration.

Nonoperative treatment is the mainstay of initial therapy and is often started before the patient presents to the orthopaedist. Primary care practitioners may have already started the patient on nonsteroidal anti-inflammatories (NSAIDs) for pain relief. In addition, patients who have rheumatoid arthritis or gout may be receiving systemic corticosteroids.

Corticosteroid injections are also an option for symptomatic relief. The duration of pain relief, however, is unpredictable and is unsubstantiated in the literature. Other injectables are also used for these conditions. Recently Salk and colleagues [19] published a pilot study of viscosupplementation for ankle arthritis. In a double blind study, 20 patients were injected with either 1 mL of sodium hyaluronate (10 mg/mL) or 1 mL of phosphate-buffered saline solution into the ankle joint. They found a significant improvement in mean ankle osteoarthritis score from baseline, but no difference between the sodium hyaluronate group and the saline group.

In addition to medications and injections, orthotic intervention can help cushion and support the arthritic subtalar and ankle joint. In general, our approach to orthoses hinges on the severity and type of deformity present. Early arthritis may get some relief with elastic inserts, sole posting, and rocker bottoms, whereas more advanced flexible deformities may benefit from nonarticulated ankle-foot orthotics, Arizona braces, or Ritchie braces. Fixed deformities need custom, well-padded orthoses that help prevent breakdown from bony prominences. In addition, some patients find relief from patellar bearing orthoses. Multiple nonoperative therapies used alone or together can significantly slow the arthritic process and provide symptomatic relief; however, these modalities cannot halt the progression.

Operative treatment

Operative intervention is often necessary in patients who have combined subtalar and ankle arthritis. Papa [8,20] found a significant number of patients who had posttraumatic arthritis and Charcot who were refractory to nonoperative intervention. These patients had frequently suffered traumatic injures with subsequent prolonged immobilization and multiple operations. Many patients also had neurologic or vascular comorbidities that complicated their clinical course. They often had debilitating pain and sequelae of their previous injuries and operations, including stiffness, atrophic skin, and vascular problems. The goal of treatment is threefold: (1) correct deformity, (2) correct instability, and (3) provide pain relief. Given the status of arthritis in patients who have failed nonoperative treatment, most operative interventions are considered salvage procedures. These include tibiotalocalcaneal (TTC) arthrodesis, total ankle arthroplasty (TAA) and subtalar fusion, Syme amputation, or below knee amputation (BKA).

Tibiotalocalcaneal arthrodesis

Tibiotalocalcaneal arthrodesis has been reported since 1911 [21]. Originally described for a flail foot, the procedure quickly gained popularity for treatment of arthritis secondary to talipes equinovarus, tuberculosis, and talus fractures [2]. Lorthioir [21] performed a procedure in which he excised the talus, denuded it, and then replaced it as a free graft. Many followed his lead using modifications to his procedure [22–24]. Leikkonen [25] was the first to mention the use of a retrograde spike placed from the calcaneus through the talus and into the tibia. This fixation was augmented by dividing the fibula and hinging it distally after denuding the cartilage surfaces. The spike was removed 10 days postoperatively. In 1956, Bingold [2] proposed arthrodesis using the fibula as a transarticular graft in seven patients. The distal 6 in of fibula were resected, the cartilage was removed, and it was passed retrograde from the calcaneus through the talus and into the tibia over a guide wire. The patient was in an above-knee cast for 4 months postoperatively. Since the advent of AO technique, ie, fracture treatment via absolute stability conferred with interfragmentary compression, there have been significant changes in these procedures; however, some similarities persist. The key concepts for managing arthritis with fusion were eloquently described by Quill [26]: (1) consider patient's age, height, and desired activity level before recommending a treatment plan, (2) fuse the painful joints, (3) fuse as few joints as possible, (4) correct deformity and maintain normal biomechanical axis in three planes, (5) provide rigid fixation for arthrodesis, (6) use bone grafts and cast immobilization if indicated, and (7) provide frequent postoperative follow-up, including rehabilitation, shoe wear selection, and restoration of the patient to the highest possible level of function.

Arthrodesis techniques

Current techniques to achieve fusion of the TTC are screws, external fixator, blade plate, or intramedullary nail. Single or combined incisions have been described, including medial, anterior, transmalleolar, and transverse approaches [7,27–31]. Screw fixation was historically the most prevalent means for achieving fusion. After the ankle and subtalar joints were exposed, the cartilage was denuded. Then the ankle was positioned at neutral DF/PF, 5° to 10° of hindfoot valgus, and external rotation that was symmetric with the contralateral side. While the ankle position was held with K-wires, bone graft was placed in the interstices. Cannulated 6.5 or 7.0 mm partially threaded cancellous screws were placed in compression across the joints. Often, two crossing screws were used from proximal anterior on the tibia to distal posterior on the calcaneus [6]. Papa and Myerson [3] described entering the heel going from posterior distal to anterior proximal passing through the subtalar joint and into the distal tibia. A second screw was placed parallel to the first with the hope that one of the two screws would capture the anterior cortex of the tibia (Figs. 3 and 4). Felix and Kitaoka [30]used a similar technique with screws placed in the opposite direction. A fibular onlay graft was often used with this technique [32]. In patients who had adequate soft tissue and bone stock, this technique worked well. Patients who had rheumatoid arthritis and diabetes, however, seemed to have problems with the fixation used in this technique. For this reason, many surgeons turned to external fixators for additional stability.

Acousta and colleagues [32] used a combination of external fixator and osseous staples to stabilize their arthrodeses (Fig. 5). They used a Calandruccio external fixation system. Russotti [5] arthrodesed 21 patients using external fixation along with a Steinman pin by way of a posterolateral approach. The joints were exposed posteriorly by splitting the Achilles tendon, the cartilage surfaces were denuded, and a trough was cut from the tibia to the calcaneus. The alignment was held by way of a retrograde Steinmann pin though the calcaneus. The Calandruccio external fixator was applied and then the trough was filled with bone graft. The external fixator was removed 9 weeks postoperatively but the Steinmann pin was retained. Russotti [5] believed the Calandruccio external fixator system to be the most effective because its biplanar stability allowed compression to be applied while the height of the hind part of the foot could be maintained simultaneously.

Hanson and Cracchiolo [33], looking for greater stability than the conventional screw techniques, turned to blade plate fixation. Using a posterior approach, he osteotomized the distal insertion of the Achilles tendon, denuded the talocrural and subtalar joints, and excised the lateral malleolus to use as bone graft with posterior iliac crest bone graft. A 95° blade plate was seated into the posterior calcaneus and secured to the distal tibia in a compression mode (Figs. 6 and 7). He believed that the posterior approach avoided incisions from previous surgery. The blade plate was especially advantageous for larger patients in whom the standard screw fixation was not adequate. Although the blade plate technique offered more stability, the approach was maximally invasive. Researchers looked for another transfixion mode that could offer stability with a less extensive approach.

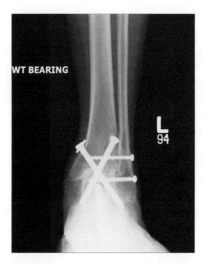

Fig. 3. Mortise radiograph of ankle with crossed screw fixation for arthrodesis.

In 1906, Lexer [34] had used a boiled cadaver bone pin as a retrograde rod. Taking a page from history, Russotti [5] started to use a larger intramedullary rod for fixation, precluded the use of an external fixator. Using a posteromedial approach instead of the trans-tendon approach, because it had fewer wound complications, the subtalar and ankle joints were exposed and denuded. An incision was made on the plantar surface of the heel and a guide wire was advanced in a retrograde fashion to the tibia. The bone was then reamed to 11.5 mm and a 12-mm intramedullary rod was inserted. The distal and plantar holes were locked with the rod flush

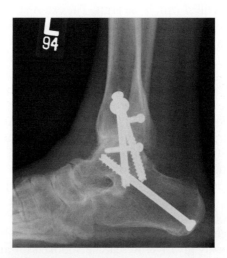

Fig. 4. Lateral radiograph of foot and ankle with crossed screw fixation for arthrodesis.

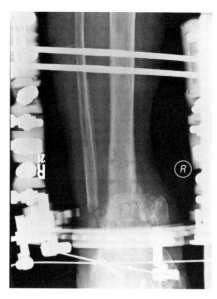

Fig. 5. AP radiograph of ankle using external fixation for arthrodesis.

to the plantar surface of the calcaneus [35]. Stephenson and colleagues [36] found that using the intersection of lines drawn from the second toe to the center of the heel in the sagittal plane and the junction of the anterior and middle thirds of the plantar heel pad in the coronal plane would give an entry point for the intramedullary rodding (IMR) that avoided damage to plantar neurovascular structures (Figs. 8 and 9). Improvement in the design of the nails continued with a posterior-to-anterior locking hole and the standard transverse holes [37]. Intramedullary fibular grafts, both vascularized

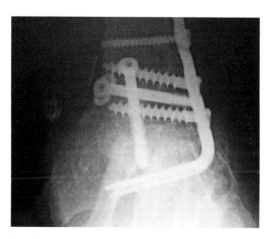

Fig. 6. AP radiograph of ankle using blade plate fixation for arthrodesis.

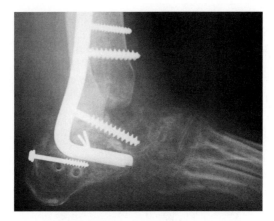

Fig. 7. Lateral radiograph of ankle using blade plate fixation for arthrodesis.

and nonvascularized, are used for the revision of intramedullary nails for arthrodesis and in situations in which there is concern regarding bony defects [38,39].

Despite the multiple procedures described for ankle and subtalar arthrodesis, obtaining fusion is still difficult in these patient populations. These patients usually have had multiple previous surgeries, skin problems, or talar viscosupplementation avascular necrosis (AVN). Also, they frequently have comorbidities, such as diabetes, and are immunocompromised secondary to medication [40]. In this setting, adjunctive measures are often

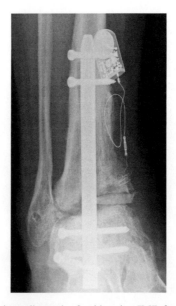

Fig. 8. Mortise radiograph of ankle using IMR for arthrodesis.

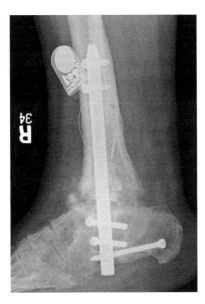

Fig. 9. Lateral radiograph of ankle using IMR for arthrodesis.

necessary to ensure union. Most procedures rely on autologous or allograft bone. In addition, many surgeons are using demineralized bone matrix on a routine basis. Donley and Ward [40] also described the use of an implantable bone stimulator for high-risk fusions. By using various bone grafts and stimulators, surgeons hope to avoid pseudoarthrosis and the need for additional revision surgery.

Postoperative management

Postoperatively, the patients who had screw and blade plate constructs were splinted or casted for 6 weeks [3,6,33], 8 weeks [8], and up to 12 weeks while remaining non–weight-bearing [30]. These patients were then transitioned to partial weight-bearing with walking casts and advanced to full weight-bearing. Patients who had intramedullary fixation were placed in short leg casts and were non–weight-bearing from 6 [34,38,41,42] to 12 weeks [4]. External fixator patients were non–weight-bearing until frame removal at 8 to 10 weeks postoperatively and subsequently placed in short-leg weight-bearing casts [5,32]. The common theme among these postoperative protocols is an initial period of non–weight-bearing to protect the fusion and hardware with gradual progression to weight-bearing as tolerated as the fusion healed.

Results

Results from the different techniques depend on the stability of the construct and the presence of fusion. Outcome from Russotti's [5] external fixator and Steinmann pin arthrodesis was 75% satisfaction and union in 18 of 21 patients. In this series, poor stability was believed to play a role in the outcome because in the 5 patients who had poor results, 2 did not have an external fixator and 2 had a Hoffman fixator that was not as stable as the Calandruccio. The fifth patient in this series had severe neuropathy that was believed to contribute to a poor outcome. Two of these 5 patients eventually went on to BKA. In another series, Acosta and colleagues [32] arthrodesed the TTC and pantalar joints in 27 feet (23 patients) using a combination of external fixation, crossed cancellous screws, and blade plates. Thirteen of 27 feet underwent TTC fusion. They found the external fixator to be unsatisfactory because of increased time to sufficient bony union (8–10 weeks), the need for extensive pin care, and need for a secondary procedure to remove the frame. In the TTC group, all patients obtained fusion, with 7 (8 feet) of 11 patients (13 feet) having good or excellent clinical results.

In 1956, Bingold [2] proposed arthrodesis using the fibula as a transarticular graft in 7 patients. All patients achieved fusion, with only 1 patient requiring a second surgery. Papa and Myerson [3] used standard screw fixation for fusion in patients who had traumatic osteoarthrosis in 21 patients. Fusion was achieved in 18 (86%); however, there were 5 (24%) malunions. Seventeen (81%) patients felt they were greatly improved, but almost all patients (20, 95%) still had residual pain. In another series, 7 patients underwent revision pantalar or TTC fusion for pseudoarthrosis with a screw construct by Levine and colleagues [6]. All achieved fusion by 14 weeks' follow-up.

Although challenges exist, fusion can be accomplished in difficult patient populations. Felix and Kitaoka [30] performed TTC fusion using screw fixation or external fixation on 12 patients who had rheumatoid arthritis (RA). All patients achieved union; however, some still reported pain. Papa and colleagues [8] performed TTC, triple, ankle, and subtalar arthrodesis using either screws or external fixation on 29 patients who had diabetic neuropathy. Some 66% (19) of the patients went on to solid union at an average of 20 weeks. There were 20 complications in 19 of the 29 patients. Pseudoarthroses were found in 10 patients, but 7 functioned well with respect to the ability to stand and walk. The total clinical stability in that study was 89%.

Stability of the crossed lag screw technique versus intramedullary rodding was examined by Bennett and colleagues [43]. They tested four different arthrodesis constructs: three crossed 6.5-mm cancellous screws, two crossed cancellous screws, locked retrograde IMR, and locked retrograde IMR with supplemental anteromedial bone staple in synthetic bone. They found that micromotion stability was best in the three cancellous screw technique. Addition of the tibiotalar staple to the IMR conferred nearly the same stability as the three-screw technique. The two-screw and IMR-only groups showed an order of magnitude less micromotion stability; however, rotation along the long axis was not tested in any of the groups. Berend and colleagues [44] tested IMR versus the crossed-screw technique in human ca-daveric bone. Twelve millimeter rods were tested in matched pairs of human cadaveric lower extremities. The biomechanical properties were compared with 6.5-mm cross-cannulated screws. They found that the IMR was signif-icantly stiffer in all four bending directions and two rotational directions.

Kile and colleagues [35] was one the first in the modern era to use a cus-tom retrograde rod for arthrodesis of the TTC. In a study of 30 patients, 84% (26) were satisfied with the outcome. Preoperative pain went from 8.3 (range 4–10) to 1.7 postoperatively (range 0–7). Three patients were dis-satisfied. Two patients were treated with BKA, and 1 experienced significant skin slough that eventually healed with a skin graft. Radiographic or clinical evidence of union was present in all but 2 patients.

Numerous articles exist in the literature that have evaluated retrograde IMR for fusion. Millet and colleagues [41] found 93% patient satisfaction and 80% return-to-work for 15 patients followed for 2 years after IMR. Mean time to union was 4 months with excellent pain relief according to An-kle-Hindfoot Scale scores. No patient had severe pain and 67% reported no pain. Hammett and colleagues [42] reviewed 52 TTC fusions performed with IMR. They found an 82% level of satisfaction with 88.5% (46/52) union achieved in an average of 4 (3–9) months. AOFAS postoperative score was 63 of 100, which is good considering 14 points of the 100 are for range of motion. Two patients went on to have amputations.

While many were performing retrograde IMR for fusion, others were us-ing a technique with potentially more stability for arthrodesis. In 2002, Han-son and Cracchiolo [33] published data regarding the use of a 95-degree blade plate for TTC fusion. Nine TTC fusions were performed using the blade plate and a posterior approach. All patients achieved solid fusion at an average of 14.7 weeks. Pain level went from moderate or severe pain daily in nine patients to no pain in five patients and mild intermittent pain in two patients. No patients had severe pain postoperatively. Complications in-cluded one episode of skin breakdown and one patient who had transient tibial nerve paresthesias. Three patients required plate removal for discom-fort at an average of 21 months postoperatively. Comparison of IMR to blade plate fixation has been done by Chiodo and colleagues [45] and Alfahd and colleagues [46]. Chiodo [45] biomechanically tested the blade plate with a 6.5-mm sagittal screw to an IMR in matched pairs of cadaveric legs. Cy-clical loading to 250,000 cycles was performed. Two specimens in the IMR group failed before the completion of the cycles. All the blade plate speci-mens completed the testing. The blade plate demonstrated significantly higher mean initial and final stiffness and decreased plastic deformation compared with the IMR fixation. The blade plate seemed to perform better, especially in osteopenic bone.

Alfahd and colleagues [46] evaluated seven matched pairs of cadaveric legs comparing IMR to a lateral cannulated blade plate construct. One plated specimen failed during testing because of screw toggle in the talus and one IMR failed. Six pairs were analyzed for angular displacement in PF, DF, inversion, eversion, internal rotation, and external rotation. No significant difference was found between the two fixations in the loading configurations. There was a small significant difference found with the blade plate internally rotated by 1.8° less than the IMR. The investigators questioned the clinical significance of this finding. They concluded that a blade plate without the sagittal screw and IMR conferred equal initial stability to the construct.

Gait

Some have expressed concern regarding the changes in gait and stress on contiguous joints attributable to TTC arthrodesis. Gellman and colleagues [14] simulated different arthrodeses in cadaveric feet and then measured the ensuing limitations of motion. Pre-arthrodesis (normal) range of motion in the ankle and foot were as follows: 27° DF, 57° PF, 29° inversion, 22° eversion, 16° hindfoot varus, and 12° hindfoot valgus. Simulated TTC fusion resulted in complete elimination of hindfoot varus and valgus. Also, DF was reduced by 53%, PF by 71%, inversion by 50%, and eversion by 48%. Pantalar fusion resulted in continued reductions. DF was reduced by 63% compared with normal, PF 82%, inversion 72%, eversion 67%. The remaining motion after TCC was largely a result of movement at Chopart's joint as evidenced by the continued reduction in movement after pantalar fusion. Ankle fusion is known to increase energy expenditure by 10% [47]. It is known that extended fusions can cause difficulty walking on uneven ground. Although there are no current biomechanical studies addressing gait after TTC, it is generally believed to cause increased stress across contiguous joints with an increase in energy expenditure during ambulation.

Arthroplasty

TAA has regained popularity because of the problems associated with fusion for arthritis. Patients who have previous subtalar fusions are more prevalent secondary to increased longevity for systemic illnesses, such as RA and lupus, and decreased mortality in patients who have extremity trauma. Ankle arthroplasty is a possible solution to concurrent ankle and hindfoot arthritis or ankle arthritis with a previous subtalar fusion. Papa [20] hypothesized that patients who have arthritic changes in the ankle joint along with subtalar or midtarsal joint arthritis may benefit from TAA because ankle arthrodesis would accelerate adjacent joint arthritis because of the abnormal loads that would be shifted from the fused ankle. AVN of the talus, which may be seen in traumatic injuries that have ankle and subtalar arthritis, is a contraindication to TAA [48]. Significant deformities cannot be corrected solely by TAA. If left uncorrected, they lead to accelerated polyethylene wear, fractures of the malleoli, and decreased time to revision [49]. TAA certainly seems to be a possible intervention for combined ankle and subtalar arthritis, but it must be used judiciously to avoid serious complications.

Complications

Numerous complications arise from interventions with combined ankle and subtalar arthritis. Some are attributable to the patient population, prior surgeries, comorbidities, and the natural history of the degenerative changes. In a study of 22 patients looking at ankle arthrodesis, there was a 14-fold increase in the rate of nonunion in smokers compared with nonsmokers [50]. Additionally, medications, such as methotrexate or prednisone, are known to affect wound healing and bone healing [50].

Complications of TTC include nonunion, malunion, infection, and soft tissue problems. Other complications include contiguous joint degeneration, nerve injury, leg length discrepancy, symptomatic hardware, and dystrophic scars. External fixators are well known for complications associated with pin tract infections, pin breakage, and decreased stability compared with other constructs [50]. Complications of IMR include wound slough, infection, malunion, delayed union, nonunion, failure of hardware, plantar foot pain at the insertion site, neurapraxia because of entry site, and stress fractures at the proximal nail junction (Figs. 10 and 11) [50–55]. Thordarson and Chang [52] found that 2 of 12 patients who had TTC fusion using an IMR had nondisplaced stress fractures at the proximal locking screws that necessitated immobilization. Biomechanical analysis of IMR revealed

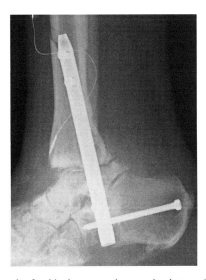

Fig. 10. Lateral radiograph of ankle demonstrating proximal stress fracture at end of IMR.

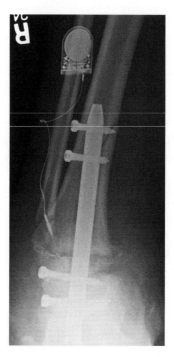

Fig. 11. AP radiograph of ankle demonstrating proximal stress fracture at end of IMR.

that standard locked nails create stress risers at the proximal screw holes. Longer retrograde rods were recommended for patients who had osteopenia [53]. Evaluation of complications after IMR revealed that patients who had diabetes had a major complication rate of 50% (including osteomyelitis, cerebral vascular accident, myocardial infarction, Charcot nonunion, loss of fixation, and full-thickness necrosis), whereas patients who did not have diabetes had no major complications [55].

Salvage of failed total ankle arthroplasty

Complications can also occur when TAA is used along with subtalar arthrodesis for treatment of combined ankle and subtalar arthritis. Complications associated with the TAA include infection, wound dehiscence, loosening, subsidence, tendon instability, and malleolar impingement [56]. Salvage can include revision and conversion to TTC arthrodesis. Kitaoka and Romness [56] revised 38 failed TAAs with TTC fusion. Eighty-nine percent union (33 of 38) was achieved. Eighty percent (24 of 38) of these patients had mild pain at an average of 8 years follow up. No patient required amputation.

Amputation

Syme or BKA is always a possible salvage for combined ankle and subtalar arthritis. It is a procedure that can allow the patient significant pain relief with a minimum of recovery time. The disadvantage to amputation is the increase in energy expenditure in a patient who may not be able to afford it. Mann [12] states, "In the end, the surgeon must realize that in certain situations, an amputation may offer the patient an expeditious and elegant solution to an otherwise severe handicap."

Summary

Combined ankle and subtalar arthritis is a difficult problem for which there are varied solutions. Each solution has its advantages and disadvantages. Treatment must be specifically tailored to the patient's needs, comorbidities, and expectations. Because of the complicated nature of this condition and its treatment, complications are common and should be anticipated.

References

[1] Hildanus GF. Observatio LXVII [letter to Dr Philibertus]. Observationum and curationum chirurgicarum centuriae. Obs 167, p. 140. Germany: Beyer. Francofurti ad Moenum 1608.

[2] Bingold AC. Ankle and subtalar fusion by a transarticular graft. J Bone Joint Surg Br 1956; 38:862–70.

[3] Papa JA, Myerson MS. Pantalar and tibiotalocalcaneal arthrodesis for post-traumatic osteoarthrosis of the ankle and hindfoot. J Bone Joint Surg Am 1992;74:1042–9.

[4] Chou LB, Mann RA, Yaszay B, et al. Tibiotalocalcaneal arthrodesis. Foot Ankle Int 2000; 21:804–8.

[5] Russotti GM, Johnson KA, Cass JR. Tibiotalocalcaneal arthrodesis for arthritis and deformity of the hind part of the foot. J Bone Joint Surg Am 1988;70:1304–7.

[6] Levine SE, Myerson MS, Lucas P, et al. Salvage of pseudoarthrosis after tibiotalar arthrodesis. Foot Ankle Int 1997;18:580–5.

[7] Shibata T, Tada K, Hashizume C. The results of arthrodesis of the ankle for leprotic neuroathropathy. J Bone Joint Surg Am 1990;72:749–56.

[8] Papa JA, Myerson MS, Girard P. Salvage, with arthrodesis in intractable diabetic neuropathic arthropathy of the foot and ankle. J Bone Joint Surg Am 1993;75:1056–66.

[9] Michelson J, Fasler M, Wigley FM, et al. Foot and ankle problems in rheumatoid arthritis. Foot Ankle Int 1994;15:608–13.

[10] Ansart MD. Pan-arthrodesis for paralytic flail. J Bone Joint Surg Br 1951;33:503–7.

[11] Bohay DR, Anderson JG. Stage IV posterior tibial tendon insufficiency: the tilted ankle. Foot Ankle Clin N Am 2003;8:619–36.

[12] Mann RA. Biomechanics of the foot and ankle. In: Mann RA, Coughlin MJ, editors. Surgery of the foot and ankle. 2nd edition. St. Louis (MO): CV Mosby; 1993. p. 3–43.

[13] Fogel GR, Katoh Y, Rand JA, et al. Talonavicular arthrodesis for isolated arthrosis: 9.5 year results and gait analysis. Foot Ankle 1982;3:105–13.

[14] Gellman H, Lenina M, Halikis N, et al. Selective tarsal arthrodesis: an in vitro analysis of the effect on foot motion. Foot Ankle 1987;8:127–33.

[15] Isman RE, Inman VT. Anthropometric studies of the human foot and ankle. In: Isman RE, Inman VT, editors. Biomechanics Lab. San Francisco, CA: University of California Technical Press; 1968.

[16] Lapidus PW. Subtalar joint: its anatomy and mechanics. Bull Hosp Jt Dis Orthop Inst 1955; 16:179–95.

[17] Mann RA. Surgical implications of biomechanics of the foot and ankle. Clin Orthop Relat Res 1980;146:111–8.

[18] Perry J. Anatomy and biomechanics of the hindfoot. Clin Orthop Relat Res 1983;177: 9–15.

[19] Salk RS, Chang TJ, D'Costa WF, et al. Sodium hyaluronate in the treatment of osteoarthritis of the ankle: a controlled, randomized, double-blind pilot study. J Bone Joint Surg Am 2006;88:295–302.

[20] Papa JA. Extended arthrodesis of the ankle and hindfoot for post-traumatic arthrosis. In: Myerson M, editor. Current therapy in foot and ankle surgery. 1st edition. St. Louis (MO): Mosby-Year Book Inc; 1993. p. 112.

[21] Lorthioir J. Huit cas d'arthrodeses du piede avec extirpation of temporaire de'lastragale. J Chir et Ann Soc Belge de Chir 1911;11:184–7 [in French].

[22] Albee FH. Bone–graft sugery. Philadelphia: W.B. Saunders Company; 1915. p. 335.

[23] Steindler A. The treatment of the flail ankle; pan-astragaloid arthrodesis. J Bone Joint Surg Am 1923;5:284.

[24] Crainz S. L'artrodesi del piede per mezzo dell'astragalectomia seguita da reimpianto parziale o totale dell'astragalo. Policlinico (Sezione Chirurgica) 1924;31:1 [in Italian].

[25] Leikkonen O. Astragaletomy as an ankle-stabilizing operation in infantile paralysis sequelae. Acta Chir Scand 1950;100:668.

[26] Quill GE. Pantalar arthritis. In: Nunley JA, Pfeffer GB, Sanders RW, et al, editors. Advanced foot and ankle reconstruction. 1st edition. Rosemont (IL): American Academy of Orthopaedic Surgeons; 2004. p. 209–14.

[27] Thordarson DB. Revision arthrodesis after failed foot and ankle surgery. Foot Ankle Clin 1996;1:13–31.

[28] Abdo RV, Wasilewski SA. Ankle arthrodesis: a long term study. Foot Ankle 1992;12: 307–12.

[29] Buratti RA, Johnson JD, Buratti D. Concurrent ankle and subtalar joint arthrodesis. J Foot Ankle Surg 1994;33:278–82.

[30] Felix NA, Kitaoka HB. Ankle arthrodesis in patients with rheumatoid arthritis. Clin Orthop Relat Res 1998;349:58–64.

[31] Holt ES, Hansen ST, Mayo KA, et al. Ankle arthrodesis using internal screw fixation. Clin Orthop Relat Res 1991;268:21–8.

[32] Acosta R, Ushiba J, Cracchiolo A. The results of a primary and staged pantalar arthrodesis and tibiotalocalcaneal arthrodesis in adult patients. Foot Ankle Int 2000;21:182–94.

[33] Hanson TW, Cracchiolo A. The use of a 95° blade plate and a posterior approach to achieve tibiotalocalcaneal arthrodesis. Foot Ankle Int 2002;23:704–10.

[34] Adams JC. Arthrodesis of the ankle joint: Experiences with the transfibular approach. J Bone Joint Surg Br 1948;30:506–11.

[35] Kile TA, Donnelly RE, Gehrke JC, et al. Tibiotalocalcaneal arthrodesis with an intramedullary device. Foot Ankle Int 1994;15:669–73.

[36] Stephenson KA, Kile TA, Graves SC. Estimating the insertion site during retrograde intramedullary tibiotalocalcaneal arthrodesis. Foot Ankle Int 1996;17:781–2.

[37] Mann MR, Parks BG, Pak SS, et al. Tibiotalocalcaneal arthrodesis: a biomechanical analysis of the rotational stability of the biomet ankle arthrodesis nail. Foot Ankle Int 2001;22: 731–3.

[38] Yajima H, Kobata Y, Tomita Y, et al. Ankle and pantalar arthrodeses using vascularized fibular grafts. Foot Ankle Int 2004;25:3–7.

[39] Ebraheim NA, Elgafy H, Stefancin JJ. Intramedullary fibular graft for tibiotalocalcaneal arthrodesis. Clin Orthop Relat Res 2001;385:165–9.

[40] Donley BG, Ward DM. Implantable electrical stimulation in high risk hindfoot fusions. Foot Ankle Int 2002;23(1):13–8.

[41] Millett PJ, O'Malley MJ, Tolo ET, et al. Tibiotalocalcaneal fusion with a retrograde intra-medullary nail: clinical and functional outcomes. Am J Orthopsychiatry 2002;531–6.

[42] Hammett R, Hepple S, Forster B, et al. Tibiotalocalcaneal (hindfoot) arthrodesis by retro-grade intramedullary nailing using a curved locking nail. The results of 52 procedures. Foot Ankle Int 2005;26:810–5.

[43] Bennett GL, Cameron B, Njus G, et al. Tibiotalocalcaneal arthrodesis: a biomechanical as-sessment of stability. Foot Ankle Int 2005;26:530–6.

[44] Berend ME, Glisson RR, Nunley JA. A biomechanical comparison of intramedullary nail and crossed lag screw fixation for tibiotalocalcaneal arthrodesis. Foot Ankle Int 1997;18:639–43.

[45] Chiodo CP, Acevedo JI, Sammarco J, et al. Intramedullary rod fixation compared with blade-plate-and-screw fixation for tibiotalocalcaneal arthrodesis: a biomechanical investiga-tion. J Bone Joint Surg Am 2003;85:2425–8.

[46] Alfahd U, Roth SE, Stephen D, et al. Biomechanical comparison of intramedullary nail and blade plate fixation for tibiotalocalcaneal arthrodesis. J Orthop Trauma 2005;19:703–8.

[47] Faillace JJ, Leopold SS, Brage ME. Extended hindfoot fusions and pantalar fusions: history, biomechanics, and clinical results. Foot Ankle Clin 2000;5:777–98.

[48] Easley ME, Vertullo CJ, Urban WC, et al. Total ankle arthroplasty. J Am Acad Orthop Surg 2002;10:157–67.

[49] Kadakia AR, Haddad SL. Ankle and hindfoot reconstruction: what is new in ankle arthro-plasty, allograft, and fusion. Curr Opin Orthop 2004;15:69–74.

[50] Cooper PS. Complications of ankle and tibiotalocalcaneal arthrodesis. Clin Orthop Relat Res 2001;391:33–44.

[51] Flock TJ, Ishikawa S, Hecht PJ, et al. Heel anatomy for retrograde tibiotalocalcaneal rod-dings: a roentgenographic and anatomic analysis. Foot Ankle Int 1997;18:233–5.

[52] Thordarson DB, Chang D. Stress fractures and tibial cortical hypertrophy after tibiotalocal-caneal arthrodesis with an intramedullary nail. Foot Ankle Int 1999;20:497–500.

[53] Noonan T, Pinzur M, Paxinos O, et al. Tibiotalocalcaneal arthrodesis with a retrograde in-tramedullary nail: a biomechanical analysis of the effect of nail length. Foot Ankle Int 2005;26:301–8.

[54] Bibbo C, Lee S, Anderson RB, et al. Limb salvage: the infected retrograde tibiotalocalcaneal intramedullary nail. Foot Ankle Int 2003;24:420–5.

[55] Mendicino RW, Catanzariti AR, Saltrick KR, et al. Tibiotalocalcaneal arthrodesis with ret-rograde intramedullary nailing. J Foot Ankle Surg 2004;43:82–6.

[56] Kitaoka HB, Romness DW. Arthrodesis for failed ankle arthroplasty. J Arthroplasty 1992;7:277–84.

ELSEVIER
SAUNDERS

Foot Ankle Clin N Am
12 (2007) 75–106

F
A

Bioadjuvants for Complex Arᴋ̣ᴜ and Hindfoot Reconstruction

Frank A. Liporace, MD[a],*, Christopher Bibbo, DO[b],
Vikrant Azad, MD[c], John Koerner, MS[d],
Sheldon S. Lin, MD[e]

[a]Department of Orthopaedic Surgery, Trauma Division,
New Jersey Medical School—University of Medicine and Dentistry New Jersey,
90 Bergen Street, Suite 1200, Newark, NJ 07103, USA
[b]Foot and Ankle Service, Department of Orthopaedics, Marshfield Clinic,
1000 North Oak Avenue, Marshfield, WI 54449, USA
[c]Department of Orthopaedic Surgery,
New Jersey Medical School—University of Medicine and Dentistry New Jersey,
90 Bergen Street, Suite 1200, Newark, NJ 07103, USA
[d]New Jersey Medical School—University of Medicine and Dentistry New Jersey,
90 Bergen Street, Suite 1200, Newark, NJ 07103, USA
[e]Department of Orthopaedic Surgery, Foot and Ankle Division,
New Jersey Medical School—University of Medicine and Dentistry New Jersey,
90 Bergen Street, Suite 1200, Newark, NJ 07103, USA

Hindfoot arthrodesis may be fraught with risks of nonunion, delayed union, malunion, infections, neuroma, avascular necrosis, and persistent pain. Overall, complication rates of up to 48% [1,2] for ankle fusion and up to 25% [3–6] for hindfoot fusion have been reported in literature.

Reconstructive options for chronic ankle and hindfoot problems include arthrodesis, arthroplasty, tendon transfers, and ligament reconstruction. Despite major advances in recent years, alternative procedures, such as total ankle arthroplasty, have not yielded consistently favorable results [7,8]. Although improvements with internal fixation devices and surgical techniques have significantly lowered the failure rate of ankle and hindfoot fusions, a substantial number of patients still suffer from nonunion [2–6,9].

* Corresponding author.
  E-mail address: frank_liporace@yahoo.com (F.A. Liporace).

1083-7515/07/$ - see front matter © 2007 Elsevier Inc. All rights reserved.
doi:10.1016/j.fcl.2006.12.002   *foot.theclinics.com*

With advances in basic science, the use of biologic adjuncts is currently being explored to supplement arthrodeses. Electrical stimulation [10,11], bone morphogenetic protein (BMP) [12,13], and platelet-rich plasma (PRP) [14–16] are some of the biologic adjuncts that have been shown to significantly enhance fusion rates. This article reviews the advances made with these technologies concerning hindfoot and ankle arthrodesis.

Arthrodesis surgeries

Triple arthrodesis

Triple arthrodesis of hindfoot involves combined fusion of subtalar, talonavicular, and calcaneocuboid joints. Triple arthrodesis remains the preferred procedure for correction of complex hindfoot deformities. Since the first description of triple arthrodesis in 1923, many triple arthrodesis techniques have been reported [17–21]. Although the results of triple arthrodesis have improved over the years, this remains a salvage procedure. The goal is to obtain a stable, painless, plantigrade foot that accommodates standard shoe wear.

Although triple arthrodesis gives reproducible results, significant complications may occur. Nonunion and pseudarthrosis have been reported as frequent causes of early failure and dissatisfaction (Table 1). Although frequently asymptomatic, the talonavicular joint is the most common site of nonunion [22,23].

Sangeorzan and colleagues [20] evaluated 40 adult patients with 44 fused feet at an average of 4.9 years after triple arthrodesis. There were 4 failures with 2 pseudarthroses and 2 unsatisfactory corrections. In a long-term review of 80 triple arthrodesis fusions followed for a mean period of 12 years, Angus and Cowell [6] reported pseudarthrosis of one or more joints in 18 feet (22%), 7 of which had significant pain with light activity. The talonavicular joint was involved in all cases of nonunion, whereas the subtalar and calcaneocuboid joints were involved in 7 of the 18 feet.

In another study Jarde and colleagues [24] reviewed 20 cases of triple arthrodesis performed for correction of adult planovalgus deformity secondary to insufficiency of the tibialis posterior tendon. Successful fusion was achieved in 18 cases. Two nonunions were reported, one affecting the talonavicular joint and the other affecting the talonavicular and calcaneocuboid joints. Results evaluated according to Kitaoka's criteria were excellent in 35%, good in 35%, fair in 20% and poor in 10% (see Table 1) [7].

Bilateral simultaneous fusions, smoking, previous infection, revision surgery, lack of rigid internal fixation, and excessive bony resection have all been reported to adversely influence union rates with triple arthrodesis.

Table 1
Clinical studies: nonunions with triple arthrodesis

References	Study	Nonunion rate	Level of evidence
Angus [6]	The results of triple arthrodesis performed in 80 feet and followed for an average of 13 years were reviewed.	Of the 79 feet pseudarthrosis of one or more joints was seen in 18 feet (22%), 7 of which had significant pain after no more than light use. The talonavicular joint was involved in all cases, other joints also in 7 of the 18.	Level IV
Sangeorzan [20]	Forty adult patients with 44 fused feet were evaluated at an average of 4.9 years after triple arthrodesis.	Thirty-four feet had good results, six had fair results, and there were four failures (two unsatisfactory corrections, two pseudarthroses).	Level IV
Jarde [24]	Review of 20 cases of valgus flatfoot deformity in the adult, secondary to insufficiency of the tibialis posterior tendon, which were treated by triple arthrodesis.	There were two nonunions: (2/20 = 10%), one affecting the talonavicular joint and the other the talonavicular and calcaneocuboid joints.	Level IV
Bennett et al [23]	Twenty-two adult patients who underwent a triple arthrodesis because of hindfoot pain and/or deformity were reviewed retrospectively with a minimum 3-year follow-up.	There were two asymptomatic nonunions of the talonavicular joint.	Level IV

Tibiotalar (ankle) fusions

The major indication for tibiotalar fusion is persistent pain attributable to end-stage arthritis of the ankle. Joint destruction secondary to various causes, such as trauma, rheumatoid arthritis, infection, or avascular necrosis of talus, culminates into arthritis of the ankle joint. The results of arthroplasty as a modality for treatment of ankle arthritis have not been as promising as in other joints, such as hip and knee, and ankle fusion is still the recommended procedure for end-stage ankle arthritis [25].

Ankle fusion also has been associated with a substantial number of complications, however, especially nonunion (Table 2). Moore and colleagues [9] published a retrospective study of retrograde intramedullary rodding for ankle arthrodesis for 19 ankles in 16 patients. Preoperative diagnoses included diabetic neuropathic arthropathy (7 patients), rheumatoid arthritis (3 patients), posttraumatic arthrosis (3 patients), paraplegia with fixed equinovarus of the foot (2 patients), and avascular necrosis of the talus (1 patient). Pseudarthrosis was seen in 5 of 19 ankles. None of the cases of pseudoarthrodesis were clinically significant, however. In another retrospective radiographic and clinical study, Anderson and colleagues [26] evaluated ankle fusions in rheumatoid arthritis patients. Ankle fusions were performed with compression screws in 35 rheumatoid ankles. Thirty-one of 35 ankles ultimately fused. Twenty-six fused with one operation resulting in a primary failure rate of 25%. Five patients required revision surgery. Twenty patients were satisfied with the result, 12 were somewhat satisfied, and 3 patients were dissatisfied.

Mann and Rongstad [25] reported the results of 81 ankle arthrodesis procedures performed by a single surgeon with 12- to 74-month follow-up. Compression screws were used for achieving fusions through the transfibular approach. Ten (12%) of the 81 ankles failed to unite. A greater resection of the medial malleolus correlated to a longer healing time and to an increased rate of nonunion. Other complications were marginal necrosis of the wound edges in 12 (15%), superficial infection in 2, and 2 major medical complications, including diabetic ketoacidosis in one and pulmonary embolism in another patient.

Frey and colleagues [2] reported on 78 ankle fusions done over 15 years. The average follow-up was 4 years. Nonunion was reported in 32 (41%) and delayed union in 9 (12%) patients. Other complications reported were infection in 7 (9%), nerve injury in 2 (3%), malunion in 2 (3%), and wound problems in 2 (3%).

Subtalar fusion

Isolated subtalar arthrodesis has been used for the treatment of numerous hindfoot problems in adults, including posttraumatic talocalcaneal arthritis [27–29], complex acute calcaneal fracture [30], primary talocalcaneal arthritis [31,32], symptomatic congenital deformity [31,32], posterior tibial tendon dysfunction [33], and inflammatory arthritis isolated to the subtalar joint. Although triple arthrodesis has been suggested for the treatment of talocalcaneal problems, advocates of isolated subtalar arthrodesis cite the advantages of preserved hindfoot motion, a lower risk for arthritis of adjacent joints, a less complex operative procedure, and elimination of the risk for nonunion or malunion of the transverse tarsal joint [31].

Various reports have shown that nonunion constitutes a significant proportion of the complications seen with isolated subtalar arthrodesis

(Table 3). In a retrospective study Trnka and colleagues [34] analyzed the results of subtalar bone block distraction arthrodesis used for the treatment of late complications of calcaneal fractures, acute severely comminuted fractures, nonunion (and malunion) of attempted subtalar arthrodeses, avascular necrosis of the talus, and club-foot deformity. Of the 37 operations, 32 (87%) achieved union and 5 went on to nonunion (13%).

In a recent large retrospective study by Easley and colleagues [35], 184 isolated subtalar fusions were reviewed to analyze the results and identify the factors influencing the union rate of isolated subtalar fusion in adults. A total of 184 subtalar arthrodeses were performed in 174 adults between 1988 and 1995. The indications for fusion included posttraumatic arthritis (after a fracture of the calcaneus [109 feet], after fracture of the talus [13 feet], or after subtalar dislocation [13 feet]), primary subtalar arthritis (13 feet), failure of a previous subtalar arthrodesis (28 feet), and residual congenital deformity (8 feet). Rigid internal fixation with one or two screws was used for all feet. Thirty patients (16%) developed nonunions. Forty-two percent (78) of the 184 feet had evidence of more than 2 mm of avascular bone at the subtalar joint. All 30 nonunions occurred in this group. The union rate in smokers was significantly less than nonsmokers (73% versus 92%). Nonunion also occurred in 3 of the 5 feet that had been treated with structural allograft and in 2 of the 6 feet in which the subtalar arthrodesis had been performed adjacent to the site of a previous ankle arthrodesis. The authors concluded that outcome following isolated subtalar arthrodesis is not as favorable as had been reported in previous studies. Factors predisposing to nonunion were smoking, the presence of more than 2 mm of avascular bone at the arthrodesis site, the use of structural allograft, and the failure of a previous subtalar arthrodesis.

Summary of foot and ankle arthrodesis

Foot and ankle arthrodeses are well-documented procedures for treating challenging clinical conditions, including posttraumatic arthritis, inflammatory arthritis, osseous defects, and Charcot arthropathy. Nonunion rates of up to 48% for ankle arthrodesis (level IV evidence) [1,2] and up to 25% for hindfoot arthrodesis (level IV evidence) [3–6] have generated concern among orthopaedic surgeons. Certain risk factors have been identified that increase delayed and nonunion rates. These risk factors include diabetes mellitus (DM), advanced age, and smoking.

Despite the paucity of literature on the impact of these risk factors on arthrodesis, the association between DM and impaired osseous healing has been examined in several level IV retrospective studies following elective arthrodesis in DM patients (level IV evidence) [36,37]. All the series noted an increased incidence (15%–30%) of delayed union, nonunion, and pseudoarthrosis (level IV evidence) [36,37]. The application of adjuncts is

Table 2
Clinical studies: nonunions with ankle arthrodesis

References	Study	Non-union	Level of evidence
Moore [9]	A retrospective study of retrograde intramedullary rodding for ankle arthrodesis in 19 ankles in 16 patients. The preoperative diagnosis of 16 patients was diabetic neuropathic arthropathy in 7 patients, rheumatoid arthritis in 3 patients, post traumatic arthrosis in 3 patients, paraplegia with fixed equinovarus of the foot in 2 patients, and avascular necrosis of the talus in 1 patient	Five of the 19 ankles (26%) had shown evidence of nonunion of arthrodesis.	Level IV
Anderson [26]	A retrospective radiographic and clinical study on 35 ankles of 35 patients for treatment of the rheumatic ankle.	31/35 ankles had healed, 26 at the first attempt and 5 after repeat arthrodesis. The primary nonunion was 9/35 (25%).	Level IV
Mann [25]	Arthrodesis of 81 ankles performed by a single surgeon reviewed after a 12- to 74-month follow-up.	Ten (12%) of the 81 ankles failed to unite.	Level IV
Primary union of ankle arthrodesis: review of a single institution/multiple surgeon experience. Dohm [104]	A review of 37 ankle arthrodesis procedures done over a 12-year period by multiple surgeons at a single institution was performed. Six different techniques were used during the study period.	The initial success rate, defined as cases achieving a solid union after the index procedure, was 65% (primary nonunion 35%). Seven additional patients went on to a solid arthrodesis after subsequent surgical procedures, for an ultimate success rate of 84%.	Level IV

(continued on next page)

Complications following arthroscopic ankle arthrodesis. Crosby [105]	Arthroscopic ankle arthrodesis in 42 patients using a biframed distraction technique and demineralized bone matrix–bone marrow slurry as a graft substitute. The average follow-up was 27 months (range, 12–64 months).	Three of 42 developed nonunion (7%)	Level IV
Frey [2]	A review of 15 years of experience with ankle fusions, specifically addressing incidence of nonunion, and associated predisposing conditions that can lead to nonunion. Seventy-eight ankle fusions, performed between 1975 and 1990, were reviewed for this study. The average follow-up was 4 years.	Delayed union in 9 (12%). Nonunion in 32 (41%).	Level IV
Ankle arthrodesis: a long-term study. Abdo [106]	This study was performed to evaluate radiographically the effect of ankle arthrodesis on tarsal motion. Thirty patients (31 ankles) were assessed for clinical and radiographic examination. The median follow-up time was 7 years (range 2–20 years)	Failed to achieve fusion in 9 patients (29%).	Level IV

Table 2 (*continued*)

References	Study	Non-union	Level of evidence
Arthrodesis of the ankle in patients who have rheumatoid arthritis. Cracchiolo [107]	A review of 32 arthrodeses of the ankle in 26 patients who had rheumatoid arthritis. In 17 patients (18 ankles), a compression arthrodesis was done and external fixation was used. In 8 patients (12 ankles), internal fixation with 6.5-mm cancellous bone screws was used. In the remaining patient, an arthrodesis with external fixation was done in one ankle and internal fixation was used in the other ankle.	Of the 19 ankles that had a compression arthrodesis, 4 failed to fuse (21%); all of the failures were associated with infection. Of the 13 ankles that had internal fixation, 3 ankles failed to fuse (23%); 1 of the failures was associated with infection.	Level IV
Long-term results of arthrodesis for osteoarthritis of the ankle. Takakura [108]	Arthrodesis in 43 joints of 42 patients who had primary and secondary osteoarthritis of the ankle. The modified anterior sliding inlay graft method was used. The average period of external immobilization was 5.8 weeks (range, 27–84 days), and follow-up ranged from 2 years 4 months to 14 years 11 months (average, 7 years 2 months)	Nonunion was detected in three (7%) patients: one patient returned to work without additional treatment; the other two patients underwent follow-up surgery within 7 months, and bony union was achieved.	Level IV
Long-term results of arthroscopic ankle arthrodesis. Ferkel [109]	Thirty-five patients with end-stage ankle arthritis underwent arthroscopic ankle arthrodesis. The average follow-up was 72 months, with a range of 24 to 167 months.	The overall fusion rate was 97% (34/35 patients). Nonunion rate of 3%.	Level IV

Table 3
Clinical studies: nonunions with subtalar arthrodesis

References	Study	Nonunion	Level of evidence
Trnka [34]	A retrospective study analyzed the results of subtalar bone block distraction arthrodesis used in the treatment of late complications of calcaneal fractures, acute severely comminuted fractures, nonunion (and malunion) of attempted subtalar arthrodeses, avascular necrosis of the talus, and club-foot deformity.	Of the 37 operations, 32 (87%) achieved union and 5 went on to nonunion (13%).	Level IV
Subtalar arthrodesis using interposition iliac crest bone graft after calcaneal fracture. Bednarz [110]	Twenty-nine feet in 28 patients who underwent subtalar distraction bone block fusion for the treatment of subtalar deformities associated with symptomatic arthrosis were evaluated.	Four nonunion.	Level IV
Easley [35]	A retrospective study to review the results of isolated subtalar arthrodesis in adults and to identify factors influencing the union rate. Between January 1988 and July 1995, 184 consecutive isolated subtalar arthrodeses were performed in 174 adults whose average age was 43 years (range, 18 to 79 years). Eighty patients (46%) were smokers. Rigid internal fixation with one or two screws was used for all feet.	Thirty feet had clinical evidence of nonunion (16%). The union rate was 84% (154/184) overall, 86% (134/156) after primary arthrodesis, and 71% (20/28) after revision arthrodesis. The union rate was 92% (93/101 feet) for nonsmokers and 73% (61/83 feet) for smokers.	Level IV

being explored for primary and revision foot and ankle arthrodesis to decrease the overall delayed and nonunion rates, especially in the at-risk groups.

Adjuncts of hindfoot arthrodesis and nonunions

Currently, a wide gamut of adjuncts exists in addition to bone grafting to facilitate a primary arthrodesis or resolve the challenging hindfoot non-union. These include internal or external bone stimulators and adjunct growth factors (ie, PRP or BMP 2).

Bone stimulators

Types of devices

Commercially, three distinct techniques exist to deliver electricity to bone in an attempt to stimulate bone healing: direct current (DC), capacitive coupling (CC), and pulsed electromagnetic field (PEMF). Direct current devices deliver electricity to bone through electrodes implanted directly on bone. Capacitive coupling devices deliver electricity to the bony area of interest through overlying skin electrodes. PEMF devices deliver electricity with the use of electromagnetic fields.

Direct current devices. DC devices are implantable devices that require the placement of a titanium cathode wire electrode in the form of a single, double, or a mesh wire directly into the fracture site with maximal surface area of contact. The battery unit houses the anode and is usually placed subcutaneously. The theoretic advantages are increased compliance, direct current application to the site of interest with maximal intensity, and constant stimulation of the osseous area of interest. Disadvantages include the need for a secondary procedure to remove the device in light of infection, local irritation, prominent hardware, and pain.

Capacitive coupling devices. Capacitance is defined as the capability of a device to store electric charge; a device designed to store charge is called a capacitor. CC devices require the placement of electrodes percutaneously over the osseous site of interest. The theoretic advantages are a more direct current application to the site of interest compared with electromagnetic field devices. Disadvantages include compliance issues secondary to long periods of use required ranging from 3 to 10 hours per day depending on the system, and local discomfort from percutaneous placement of electrodes.

Pulsed electromagnetic field devices. PEMF devices use the local application of pulses of electricity delivered to the area of interest in the form of an electromagnetic field. Advantages of PEMF devices include their noninvasive nature and their ability to be worn directly on the skin or a cast. Long periods of use are recommended by the manufacturers, ranging from 3 to 10 hours per day depending on the system. Compliance is thus a major issue. Use of PEMF devices less than the recommended minimum period of 3 hours has been demonstrated to significantly reduce the efficacy of this modality of bone stimulation in union rates, with approximately 2.3 times less union reported compared with when PEMF is used for the recommended period of time (level III evidence) [38].

In vitro studies—potential mechanisms

Previous in vitro studies have attempted to elucidate the mechanisms of action for PEMF, DC, and CC fields (Table 4). PEMF seems to stimulate healing of a nonunion through the differentiation of fibrocartilage cells mediated by TGF-β expression [39]. The stimulatory effect of PEMF on osteoblasts seems to be mediated through up-regulation of BMP-2 and BMP-4 expression in addition to an increase in calcium uptake induced by nitric oxide synthase [40–42]. The stage at which PEMF stimulation acts has produced conflicting data regarding proliferation and differentiation. DC seems to stimulate bone formation through an increase in intracellular free calcium and hydrogen peroxide generation at the cathode and the resulting increase in pH [43,44]. CC increases osteoblast proliferation induced by an increase in TGF-β expression through activation of the calcium/calmodulin pathway [45,46].

Does PEMF treatment promote bone healing in a nonunion model?

In a rat fibula model, bilateral 6-mm osteotomies were allowed to reach a nonunion state until 28 days postsurgery [47]. At this point, a PEMF waveform (pulse frequency of 3.8 kHz, maximum amplitude of ~2 mT)

Table 4
Clinically available electric bone stimulation devices

Manufacturer/device name	Type of device	Recommended application time	Recommended indications
EBI Bone Healing System	PEMF	10 h/d	Nonunions, failed fusions, congenital pseudoarthrosis
EBI OstroGen	DC	24 h/d	Nonunions
Biolectron OrthoPak	CC	24 h/d	Nonunions
Physio-Stim Lite (OrthoFix)	PEMF	3 h/d	Nonunions
DonJoy OL1000 (Orthologic)	PEMF	30 min/d	Nonunions

Data from Kesani AK, Gandhi A, Lin SS. Electrical bone stimulation devices in foot and ankle surgery: types of devices, scientific basis, and clinical indications for their use. Foot Ankle Int 2006;27(2):148–56.

was applied for 3 hours daily for 10 weeks. PEMF treatment demonstrated a significant reduction in the amount of time-dependent bone volume loss in the distal fibular segments. In addition, the osteotomy gap size was significantly smaller in hind limbs exposed to PEMF.

In a canine tibia osteotomy gap model simulating delayed healing, PEMF treatment (pulse frequency of 1.5 Hz, maximum amplitude ~ 2 G) was initiated four weeks postsurgery for a total of 8 weeks [48]. PEMF treated osteotomies demonstrated faster recovery of dynamic load bearing with increased load-bearing capacity compared with the untreated group. The biomechanical properties of the healing osteotomy were significantly greater in the PEMF-treated group.

Indications for use of bone stimulators and supporting clinical evidence

Review of the electrical bone stimulation device literature demonstrates several clinical trials and studies demonstrating its beneficial effects on bone healing in the lower extremity. These studies vary greatly in study design and quality, however. The authors use the Level of Evidence and Grades of Recommendation table developed by the American Academy of Orthopaedic Surgeons (AAOS) to classify the available clinical studies (Box 1).

Box 1. Level of evidence and grades of recommendation

Level of evidence
Level I: high-quality prospective randomized clinical trial
Level II: prospective comparative study
Level III: retrospective case control study
Level IV: case series
Level V: expert opinion

Grades of recommendation (given to various treatment option based on level of evidence supporting that treatment)
Grade A: treatment options are supported by strong evidence (consistent with level I or II studies)
Grade B: treatment option are supported by fair evidence (consistent with level III or IV studies)
Grade C: treatment option are supported by either conflicting or poor-quality evidence (level IV studies)
Grade I: insufficient evidence exist to make a recommendation

---

Data from Kesani AK, Gandhi A, Lin SS. Electrical bone stimulation devices in foot and ankle surgery: types of devices, scientific basis, and clinical indications for their use. Foot Ankle Int 2006;27(2):148–56.

Foot and ankle arthrodesis

Foot and ankle arthrodeses are commonly performed procedures to deal with various pathologic processes; however, the fusion rates are less than desirable. Electrical bone stimulation has been considered for primary and revision foot and ankle arthrodesis to improve clinical results and minimize complications (Table 5).

Primary arthrodesis

Examination of the literature demonstrates one level I PEMF study [10] and two level IV DC studies [49,50] demonstrating the beneficial effect of electrostimulation in the treatment of primary hindfoot fusions (see Table 5).

Dhawan and colleagues [10] reported a level I prospective randomized clinical trial evaluating PEMF. A total of 64 patients (144 joints) underwent elective triple or isolated hindfoot arthrodesis for primary and revision surgery. Radiographic analysis using a blinded musculoskeletal radiologist revealed a statistically significant reduction in time required for union in the talonavicular and calcaneocuboid fusions in PEMF-treated group, and a trend toward faster union rate in the subtalar arthrodesis group. The control group average time to union was 14.5 weeks in 33 primary subtalar fusions with 4 nonunions, 17.6 weeks in 19 primary talonavicular fusions, and 17.7 weeks in 21 primary calcaneocuboid fusions with 1 nonunion. The PEMF-treated group's average time to union was 12.9 weeks in 22 primary subtalar fusions, 12.2 weeks in talonavicular fusions, and 13.1 weeks in calcaneocuboid fusions. No patients in the PEMF group developed a nonunion. In those patients who underwent PEMF treatment of multiple joint arthrodeses there was a tendency for the remaining joints to fuse more quickly when one of the joints fused rapidly. The study excluded patients considered high risk, specifically those who had rheumatoid arthritis, diabetes, or corticosteroid use, which decreases the strength of the study. Additionally, no sham PEMF units for controls were used, and the risk factor data was not reported.

The DC stimulation studies included two level IV case series analyzing foot and ankle arthrodeses. A somewhat lower rate of union (65%) was noted compared with other series using the implantable bone stimulation device. Lau and colleagues [50] attributed this low rate to the characteristics of the patients. All patients had at least two risk factors for nonunion and 35% were revision procedures. A complication rate of 35% (excluding nonunions) included deep infection of the implant, deep venous thrombosis, wound breakdown, and one amputation for recalcitrant neuroma. A 15% rate of deep infection of the implant occurred in high-risk patients, specifically in patients who smoked or who had diabetic Charcot arthropathy. Overall, 78% of patients were functionally improved and 89% achieved a satisfactory result. The authors concluded that the use of implantable DC stimulators is reasonable with an acceptable complication rate in these high-risk groups.

Table 5
Clinical evidence for electrical stimulation on delayed union/non-union

Study	Study level	No. of patients	Bone stimulator type	Outcome (% fusion rates or average healing times)
Sharrard et al, 1990 {Sharrard, 1990 #1124}	I	20 Rx 25 C	PEMF	45% fusion in treatment group, 12% fusion in control group
Scott et al, 1994 {Scott, 1994 #1123}	I	10 Rx 11 C	CC	60% fusion in treatment group, 0% fusion in control group
de Haas et al, 1980 {de Haas, 1986 #1092}	III	17 Rx 23 C	PEMF	88.2% fusion in treatment group, 82.5% in control group
Holmes et al, 1994 {Holmes, 1994 #1105}	IV	9 Rx	PEMF	Average healing time of 3 months
Heckman et al, 1990 {Heckman, 1981 #1104}	IV	149 Rx	PEMF	64.4% fusion in treatment group
Paterson et al, 1980 {Paterson, 1980 #1118}	IV	8 Rx	DC	86% fusion in treatment group
Brighton et al, 1981 {Brighton, 1985 #1085}	IV	175 Rx	DC	83.7% fusion in treatment group

Abbreviations: C, control group; Rx, treatment group.
Data from Kesani AK, Gandhi A, Lin SS. Electrical bone stimulation devices in foot and ankle surgery: types of devices, scientific basis, and clinical indications for their use. Foot Ankle Int 2006;27(2):148–56.

The other DC level IV study, performed by Donley and Ward [49], consisted of 13 patients with an average follow-up of 24.6 months. Patients had hindfoot or ankle fusions (6 tibiotalocalcaneal, 3 ankle, 2 subtalar, and 2 tibiocalcaneal arthrodeses) augmented with DC bone stimulation. All had at least two risk factors for nonunion, including history of nonunion, smoking, or avascular necrosis of the talus. Twelve patients had achieved a successful fusion. Statistically significant improvement was achieved at 1 year compared with preoperative scores using modified American Orthopaedic Foot and Ankle Society (AOFAS) scoring system. The only reported complication was a superficial wound breakdown treated successfully by intravenous antibiotics. Four reoperations for removal of the batteries were noted.

Because of the paucity of literature evaluating PEMF and DC bone stimulation with hindfoot and ankle arthrodesis, it is difficult to define its role. Sufficient clinical evidence does not exist to support the use of invasive DC devices over noninvasive PEMF devices.

Revision arthrodesis

Foot and ankle arthrodesis revision procedures pose a high nonunion risk. As a result, considerable interest has been generated regarding the application of electrostimulation to revision arthrodeses. Despite this well-known clinical challenge, few studies exist. Only one level IV DC study [51] exists demonstrating the beneficial effects and one level IV PEMF study [11] demonstrating poor results of electrostimulation on revision arthrodeses (Table 6). Midis and Conti [51] performed a level IV case series analyzing 10 consecutive revision arthrodeses for patients who had aseptic nonunion of the ankle using DC bone stimulation. All of their patients obtained solid bony union at an average of 12.8 weeks. The modified AOFAS scores showed 70% good to excellent results.

In contrast, Saltzman and colleagues [11] performed a level IV retrospective case series on a series of nonunions after foot and ankle arthrodesis. In 334 foot and ankle arthrodeses, they noted 19 delayed unions, using a protocol with PEMF, immobilization, and limited weight bearing. Only 26% (5/19 patients) of the nonunions were successfully treated with this method. Sixty-four percent (9/14) of the subsequent nonunion group had revision surgery with a similar fusion rate of 22% (2/9 patients). Patient risk factors included smoking (5 patients) and previous nonunions (8 patients). The authors did not recommend immobilization and PEMF as a protocol for treating delayed union in foot and ankle arthrodesis and hypothesized that the mechanical difficulties in orienting the coils around the foot and ankle may partially explain the lower success compared with long bones.

In view of the limited number of level IV studies (one level IV DC and one level IV PEMF study) demonstrating an inconsistent influence of electrical bone stimulation on the foot and ankle revision arthrodeses, the routine use of electrical bone stimulation in this scenario is difficult to justify (grade C). Furthermore, contrary to the previous indications, limited data

Table 6
Clinical evidence for foot and ankle arthrodesis

Study	Study level	No. of patients in treatment group	Bone stimulator type	Outcome (% fusion rates or average healing times)
Arthrodesis primary				
Dhawan et al [10]	I	144	PEMF	TN, faster with PEMF CC, faster with PEMF ST, no difference
Lau et al [50]	IV	40	DC	65% fusion in treatment group
Donley et al [49]	IV	13	DC	92% fusion in treatment group
Revision arthrodesis				
Midis et al [51]	IV	10	DC	Average healing time of 12.8 weeks
Saltzman et al [11]	IV	19	PEMF	26% fusion in treatment group

Abbreviations: CC, calcaneocuboid; ST, subtalar; TN, talonavicular.

Data from Kesani AK, Gandhi A, Lin SS. Electrical bone stimulation devices in foot and ankle surgery: types of devices, scientific basis, and clinical indications for their use. Foot Ankle Int 2006;27(2):148–56.

exist to support the use of DC devices over PEMF devices for revision arthrodesis.

Summary

Although there is evidence that is suggestive of electrostimulation being beneficial for increasing foot and ankle arthrodesis union rates, insufficient evidence exists for supporting the routine use of electrostimulation with foot and ankle arthrodesis. Furthermore, little peer-reviewed scientific literature exists to justify its routine use for treatment of high-risk fresh fractures, such as tibia and metaphyseal-diaphyseal fifth metatarsal fractures of the foot. Further prospective randomized controlled studies are needed to justify its use for this indication.

Platelet-rich plasma

PRP, derived from autologous blood, is defined as a volume of plasma that has a platelet concentration that is typically a fivefold increase ($\sim$1,000,000/mL) above physiologic levels. PRP serves as a reservoir of critical growth factors, including platelet-derived growth factor (PDGF), TGF-β, and insulin-like growth factor–I (IGF-I). Although there is an abundance of literature pertaining to dental applications, this review highlights the use of PRP in orthopaedic applications ranging from PRP preparation to in vitro and in vivo studies to clinical research.

Introduction of concept of critical growth factors

At the site of any trauma involving bone, a clot forms consisting of red blood cells, white blood cells, and platelets entrapped within a fibrin matrix. In the bone repair process, the platelet α-granules act as a reservoir of exogenous growth factors. The degranulation of the α-granules results in the release of PDGF, IGF, and TGF-β among a host of other growth factors providing an ideal delivery system localized to the site of injury. Each of these factors plays a critical role in bone healing.

PDGF enhances DNA synthesis, increases collagen deposition, and stimulates synthesis of extracellular matrix [52]. In vitro, PDGF has been shown to stimulate type I collagen production and mRNA expression in osteoblasts and chondrocytes [53]. PDGF has enhanced chemotactic and proliferative effects and the ability to initiate differentiation of osteoprogenitor cells toward an osteoblastic lineage [54]. PDGF functions in a macrophage autocrine feedback loop stimulating production and release of growth factors or cytokines [55].

Joyce and colleagues [53] analyzed the effect of daily injection of PDGF into uninjured newborn rat femurs. Their findings suggest that PDGF initiated osteogenesis and chondrogenesis. Daily injections of PDGF resulted in a dose-dependent increase in mesenchymal cell proliferation with a mass of new bone formation. In a unilateral rabbit tibial osteotomy model, the application of exogenous PDGF exhibited a stimulatory effect on bone healing [56]. Fujii and colleagues [57] analyzed the expression of PDGF along with α- and β-receptor mRNA to further elucidate its role in the inflammatory phase (days 2–4) after fracture. These investigators theorized that the function mediated by the β receptor, including cell migration, might be prerequisite to the recruitment of mesenchymal cells in the initial step and to the interaction between osteoclasts and osteoblasts in the bone remodeling phase.

IGF seems to play a critical role in skeletal development by stimulating osteoblastic cell proliferation and differentiation as a function of the stage of cell maturation [58]. IGF-I stimulates proliferation of osteoblast precursors and early-stage osteoblasts and promotes bone matrix formation by fully differentiated osteoblasts [59–63]. IGF-I stimulates type I collagen and noncollagenous matrix protein synthesis in bone cultures independently of their mitogenic activity. In addition, IGF inhibits collagen degradation by way of inhibition of collagenase expression by osteoblasts [59]. Mochizuki and colleagues [64] reported that IGF-I stimulated bone resorption by pre-existing osteoclasts. Hill and colleagues [65] suggested that osteoblasts mediate this IGF-I stimulation of osteoclast activation because they found no stimulation of isolated osteoclast activity unless osteoblasts were present. IGF has been shown to be expressed by the primary cultures of rat osteoblasts and by transformed and osteosarcoma-derived osteoblastic cell lines [66]. The stage of osteoblast differentiation seems to influence the pattern of IGF expression. In fetal rat calvarial cultures, IGF-I secretion has been shown to be biphasic. Early-stage IGF expression was associated with cell proliferation. As preosteoblasts differentiated, IGF-I secretion decreased, with a second increase occurring late during mineralization [67].

In vivo, endogenous and exogenous IGF has been associated with indices of active bone matrix production [68–70]. IGF expression has also been found to be the highest in osteoblasts that are involved in active bone remodeling [70]. Similarly, Middleton and colleagues [69] and Andrew and colleagues [68] demonstrated in adult human osteophyte tissue and normally healing human fracture, respectively, that IGF-I expression was strongest in osteoblasts actively forming bone and weak or absent in quiescent flat bone lining cells and in osteocytes. Analysis of temporal aspects of IGF expression during rat bone formation (induced by implantation of demineralized bone matrix) indicated a transient increase in IGF-I mRNA occurring at day 3 associated with proliferation of osteoblastic cells. After a tibia fracture, IGF-I mRNA in the rat fracture callus increased over time and peaked on day 8 with a 10- to 15-fold increase compared with control bone [71].

Another growth factor of importance in the early stage of fracture healing is TGF-β. There is nearly 100% sequence conservation across mammalian species. It is secreted as an inactive or latent complex. Activation and cleavage to the mature peptide occurs through an unknown enzymatic reaction. Bone and platelets contain almost 100 times more TGF-β than any other tissue and osteoblasts have the highest number of TGF-β receptors [72,73]. These findings suggest that TGF-β plays a key role in bone metabolism.

In rat calvarial and human osteoblasts and corresponding cell lines, TGF-β increased cell proliferation [74,75]. Both collagen production and gene expression can be stimulated by TGF-β [76,77]. In a fracture callus organ explant culture, exogenous application of TGF-β stimulated type I collagen and osteonectin production and also increased DNA synthesis by twofold [78]. TGF-β has the ability to stimulate differentiation of mesenchymal cells into cells with a chondrocytic phenotype [79] and the synthesis of type II collagen and proteoglycans by mesenchymal cells [80], suggesting a role for TGF-β in regulating chondrocyte differentiation and cartilage matrix production.

These aforementioned studies suggest that the growth factors (PDGF, IGF, and TGF-β) contained within platelets that are present at the site of injury play a critical role in the healing process. The delivery of increased levels of these critical growth factors is accomplished by producing PRP. An important biologic corollary of platelet function in bone healing was elucidated by Babbush and colleagues [81]. The investigators demonstrated that PDGF and TGF-β concentrations were linearly correlated to the number platelets. PRP has been defined as a volume of plasma that has a platelet concentration greater than physiologic levels, typically a fivefold increase.

In vitro studies

In addition to the demonstrated chemoattractive and proliferative effects of PRP, an in vitro study sought to demonstrate the effect of PRP on osteoblast differentiation [82]. PRP was prepared from human volunteers that concentrated platelets by 344% compared with venous blood. After 24 hours PRP enhanced ALP activity in a time-dependent manner compared with platelet-poor plasma. Procollagen type I expression and osteopontin expression also increased with increasing PRP concentration. Osteopontin expression showed a similar trend during the growth phase and at confluence osteopontin expression was detected only with 10% PRP. During the growth phase, PRP had no effect on osteoprotegerin expression but at confluence, osteoprotegerin expression was detected only with 10% PRP. At confluence, cbfa1 expression was detected only with 10% PRP. These results suggest that osteoblast-like cells undergoing proliferation have suppressed differentiation. At confluence, however, PRP-enhanced expression of genes responsible for osteoblast growth and differentiation.

Clinical applications and current results of platelet-rich plasma in hindfoot arthrodesis

The mechanism of action of PRP that involves platelet degranulation, the release of various growth factors, and subsequent stimulation of stem cell lines is complex. Currently, there is a paucity of clinical data in the orthopaedic literature regarding outcomes with the use of PRP.

One of the first reports (level IV) of the use of PRP in foot and ankle patients was by Gandhi and colleagues [83]. This preliminary study centered on the use of PRP in nine patients who had sustained a foot and ankle nonunion. In this Institutional Review Board-approved prospective study, all patients had undergone initial surgical intervention performed within 20 days of their foot and ankle fracture. All of these patients were diagnosed with a nonunion for a minimum duration of 4 months. Their revision treatment operation was the focus of this study. This study population possessed a nonunion of 4 to 10 months' duration after diagnosis; the mean patient age was 42 years. The authors applied PRP and autogenous bone graft to the nonunion site along with standard fixation techniques. Their findings indicated that, with the addition of PRP and bone graft, resolution of a nonunion was achieved at a mean time of 60 days. Within this study, Gandhi and colleagues compared growth factor concentrations at the surgical site within the fracture hematoma in patients who had a nonunion versus patients who did not have a nonunion. In examining growth factor levels, plasma levels of PDGF and TGF-β were consistent between patients with a nonunion versus fresh fracture. A significant reduction was noted in growth factor levels in the fracture hematoma levels versus nonunion site in patients who had a nonunion versus fresh fracture. This study clearly implicates that the local milieu in fresh fractures versus those that have gone on to a nonunion exhibits a significant difference in these important bone-healing factors. The addition of PRP and the subsequent release of platelet-associated growth factors may provide critical early growth factors to the nonunion site resulting in a positive impact on resolving nonunions.

The first published evidence-based study on the use of PRP in foot and ankle surgery was published by Bibbo and colleagues [16]. In this level II study the investigators examined the clinical results and complications of the adjuvant use of PRP in high-risk patients undergoing elective foot and ankle surgery. High-risk patients were enrolled over a 6-month period in this prospective, intention-to-treat study. Investigation involved 62 patients, which encompassed 123 operative procedures, the vast majority involving fusions. The mean patient age was 51 years, ranging from 16 to 76, with a slight preponderance of women. The study inclusion criteria included patients who had risk factors for bone healing difficulties (ie, 37% of patients were smokers, 11% of patients had diabetes). More than 69% of study patients had multiple risk factors. In this study, patients received bone graft only when required to fill a bone defect or to correct alignment (eg, lateral column lengthening). The addition of autograft did not seem to have any significant improvement in fusion rate. Overall, there was a 94% union rate in the foot and ankle with a mean time to union of 41 days (Table 7).

Among the patients who went on to nonunion, all four patients developed an infection. Infections incurred in patients who had diabetes, Charcot arthropathy, and skin ulcerations, and patients who had a collagen vascular disorder. In some instances, infection occurred after a surgical site had radiographically seemed to proceed on to union, with secondary infection after a delay in wound healing. The authors of this study concluded that the adjunctive use of PRP is an important tool in high-risk elective foot and ankle surgery whether a bone graft is used or not, resulting in an acceptable time to union with low risk for complications. The authors also briefly compared their results to those of implantable DC stimulators. The results of the PRP series provided an improved time to union and an increased union rate with a lower complication rate than that associated with implantable DC stimulators.

Two articles have been published within the past year focusing on the distal tibia-fibular syndesmotic fusion site and the role of PRP. Barrow and Pomeroy [84] reported their level IV study analyzing the role of PRP in primary distal tibia-fibular syndesmotic fusion. As part of the distal tibia-fibula fusion of total ankle replacement, autologous platelet concentrate was used at the distal tibia-fibular fusion site in 20 consecutive total ankle replacements. The fusion rate was 100%. Similarly, a level III study performed by Coetzee and colleagues [14] examined the application of PRP in foot and ankle surgery also excerpted from a larger study on Agility total ankle replacement (TAR) (Depuy, Inc., Warsaw, IN). In this study, the authors compared syndesmotic fusion rates using PRP-augmented bone grafting versus historical control of non-PRP–augmented bone grafting of

Table 7
Time to union by anatomic region and use of bone graft

Anatomic region	Mean time to union with PRP (d)[a]			Mean all groups (auto + allo + no graft) (n = 123)	Overall union rate
	Autograft (n = 46)	Allograft (n = 10)	No bone graft (n = 67)		
Ankle (n = 21)	43 (1 nonunion)	31	43	40	95%
Hindfoot (n = 26)	48 (2 nonunion)	—[b]	39	43	92%
Midfoot (n = 66)	46 (2 nonunion)	30	41 (2 nonunion)	41	94%
Forefoot (n = 10)	45	—[b]	30	38	100%
Σ (N = 123)	45[c]	31	40[c]	41	94%

[a] Days rounded to nearest whole number.
[b] Graft not used in this category.
[c] $P = .0173$, two-tailed t-test; no statistical difference in mean time to union with the addition of autograft to PRP.

Data from Bibbo C, Bono CM, Lin SS. Union rates using autologous platelet concentrate alone and with bone graft in high-risk foot and ankle surgery patients. J Surg Orthop Adv 2005;14(1):17–22.

the ankle syndesmosis performed during TAR surgery. Their study compared 66 patients to 114 historical controls. Union was analyzed prospectively by radiographs and CT. The investigators found, among their historical controls of syndesmotic fusions with bone graft alone, a 61% fusion rate was achieved at 8 weeks, a 73% fusion rate at 12 weeks, and an 85% fusion rate at 6 months. In contrast, syndesmotic fusion rates during TAR using PRP with bone graft resulted in a 76% union rate at 8 weeks, 94% union rate at 3 months, and 97% union rate at 6 months. A statistically significant improvement in the time to union and overall union rate was seen at 8 and 12 weeks. It is also important to note that among this study group a high-risk subset of smokers achieved a 50% union rate at 6 months in the control group and 80% in the PRP and bone graft group. The data demonstrated PRP, in this clinical setting, improves the time to union in ankle syndesmotic fusions, which is a critical next step required before patients can proceed with advanced weight-bearing status and the overall success of the Agility TAR.

The evolving role of bone morphogenetic proteins and potential future applications

The formation of a sound arthrodesis requires the terminal ends of two bones to be denuded of intervening cartilage and fibrous tissue. Through stable fixation, the bone ends are approximated and the goal of healing two bones together commences. This situation is analogous to operative fracture management through open reduction, acquisition of appropriate alignment of bone fragments, and stable fixation. Both situations require the appropriate biologic milieu to allow for the steps of bone healing.

Bone healing occurs through a specific order of events. It commences with hematoma and a local inflammatory reaction that induces the invasion of neutrophils and monocytes for removal of cellular debris and degradation of fibrin clot. Then revascularization with invasion of blood vessels occurs. Next, cellular proliferation with multiplication of proliferative connective tissue progenitor cells occurs. Subsequently, a matrix synthesis occurs that causes initial differentiation of progenitor cells. Cellular differentiation is based on many factors, including oxygen tension and mechanical stimuli. With high strain, fibrous tissue is produced. With low strain and high oxygen tension, woven bone forms by way of intramembranous ossification. Intermediate strain and low oxygen tension induce cartilage formation. As strain conditions improve, endochondral ossification occurs and bone replaces cartilage. Finally, remodeling occurs. Osteoclastic and chondroclastic resorption allow for subsequent replacement with mature lamellar bone [85–87].

The formation of bone relies on osteogenesis, osteoinduction, and osteoconduction. Osteogenesis is the ability of grafted cells to form bone by way of osteoblastic stem cells and progenitor cells. Osteoinductivity is the ability to modulate the differentiation of stem cells and progenitor cells along an osteoblastic pathway. Osteoconductivity is the ability to provide the scaffold for new bone to be laid down. These processes are mediated by multiple cytokines, including BMP.

BMPs, except BMP 1, are members of the TGF superfamily and have regulatory effects in the differentiation of cartilage and bone-forming cells from pluripotential mesenchymal cells during the processes of bone healing [85]. During these processes, PDGF, TGF-β, and BMPs are expressed. BMPs are osteoinductive and promote cellular proliferation, apoptosis, differentiation, and morphogenesis. They induce bone formation by way of endochondral ossification and in high concentrations may form bone by way of intramembranous ossification [88]. They are key modulators of osteoprogenitor and mesenchymal cells during fracture healing. Rat studies have shown that chondrocytes and osteoblasts exhibit increased expression of BMP. BMP 2 and 4 seem to drive osteoprogenitor cells to mature into osteoblasts [89]. BMP 2 concentrations have been shown to be elevated as early as the hematoma phase. BMPs 3a, 4, and 7 increase concentrations later in the osteogenic phase when bone maturation commences [90–92]. As precursor cells mature and callus remodels, BMP 2 expression decreases [87]. More than 20 BMPs have been identified. BMP 2, 4, and 7 seem to have the most prominent role in bone formation [93]. Commercially available BMPs include BMP 2 and 7.

In vitro studies have shown that BMP 2 and 7 facilitate healing critical-sized defects [87,94,95]. In a rat femur model with a segmental defect, Yasko and colleagues [95] showed BMP 2 induced a 100% union rate. Bouxsein and colleagues [96] demonstrated that BMP 2 could induce healing in a rabbit ulna osteotomy model. Most importantly, the investigators demonstrated that specimens treated with BMP 2 had an 80% increase in torsional strength after 3 weeks compared with specimens not treated with BMP 2. By 4 weeks, the specimens treated with BMP 2 were biomechanically equivalent to intact ulna, whereas the controls were only 45% as strong. Through quantitative computed tomography, the authors demonstrated that the BMP 2–treated specimens had a 60% increase in the area of mineral content at 3 weeks of healing.

In fracture healing and spinal fusions, BMPs have been shown to be beneficial. In a prospective randomized clinical trial, 450 patients who had open tibia fractures were randomized to receive intramedullary nailing (IMN), or IMN with one of two doses of BMP 2. Compared with patients who received solely IMN, those who also received high-dose BMP 2 had significantly fewer hardware failures, shorter time to union, fewer infections, faster wound healing, and fewer nonunions [97].

The use of BMPs has also been shown help with nonunion surgery. A recent series of 12 patients who had femoral nonunions had a 100% union rate at 5 months when BMP was used to supplement revision surgery. Patients had averaged four prior surgeries each for treatment of their femur fractures before receiving BMP [98]. Friedlaender and colleagues [99] evaluated 124 tibial nonunions in a prospective, randomized, multicenter trial. Patients were treated with IMN and autograft or IMN and BMP 7 with a collagen carrier. At 9 months, 81% of the BMP 7–treated group and 85% of the autograft group exhibited clinical healing. By 2 years of observation, there were no statistically significant differences in outcome between the two groups. Greater than 20% of patients treated with autograft had chronic donor site pain.

BMPs have been used as adjuncts or substitutes to bone grafting in posterior spinal fusions. A recent study showed that mesenchymal stem cells genetically engineered to express BMP 2 could induce bone formation in paraspinal muscles of mice. The authors demonstrated that genetically engineered mesenchymal stem cells induce bone formation in areas adjacent to and touching the posterior elements of the spine by way of induction of active osteogenesis at the site of implantation for up to 4 weeks postinjection [100]. Clinically, a recent randomized prospective trial showed that anterior spinal fusion patients who received allograft and BMP 2 had decreased length of surgery, less blood loss, shorter hospital stays, significantly higher fusion rates, and higher SF-36 scores than patients who underwent fusion with autograft [101].

The questions of dose-related response of BMP and the possibility of synergy have recently been explored. David and colleagues have shown in a canine spinal fusion model that BMP 2 has a dose-dependent osteoinductive effect [102]. It has also been proposed that the combination of BMP 2 and 7 could induce greater effects than either alone [103]. In a posterolateral rat spine fusion model, use of BMP 2 and 7 together induced a significantly greater expression of osteocalcin and ALP and greater mineralization and higher bone volume than using either alone [104].

Case examples of bone morphogenetic protein use in hindfoot and ankle fusions

In 2000, OP-1 (BMP 7) received a Humanitarian Device Exemption approval from the Food and Drug Administration for the treatment of recalcitrant nonunions of long bones. Extrapolating from this, we present two cases using BMP as an adjunct in at-risk hindfoot and ankle fusions.

Case 1. A 57-year-old obese woman was referred with a chief complaint of severe hindfoot pain with ambulation approximately 1 year after open reduction with internal fixation (ORIF) of an intra-articular calcaneus fracture. She had delayed wound healing after ORIF. Evaluation of the patient revealed severe subtalar arthrosis, best appreciated on CT (Fig. 1A). A subtalar fusion was planned. Preoperatively, the patient was on chronic nonsteroidal anti-inflammatory drug therapy and had undergone a series of corticosteroid injections, placing her at risk for nonunion. At surgery, a posterior approach to the subtalar joint was selected. Percutaneous removal of the plate and screws was attempted, but the screw heads were

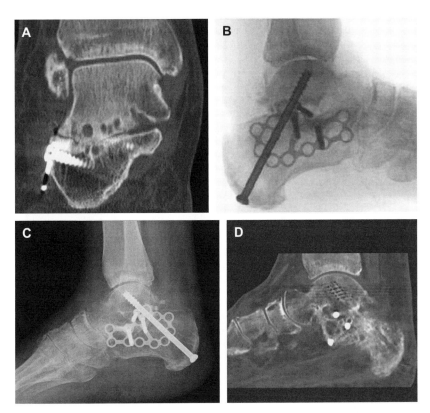

Fig. 1. (*A*) Coronal CT scan image displaying posttraumatic subtalar arthrosis in a patient who had an intra-articular calcaneus fracture. (*B*) Intraoperative fluoroscopic lateral image demonstrating subtalar fusion augmented with BMP 2. (*C*) Lateral radiograph displaying bony union of subtalar fusion at 12 weeks. (*D*) Sagittal CT scan image displaying bony union of subtalar fusion at 12 weeks.

stripped. Because of her poor wound-healing history, extension of the incision to remove her hardware was not performed. Rigid screw fixation of subtalar joint fusion was augmented with rhBMP-2 (Fig. 1B). An uncomplicated postoperative course was followed by radiographic fusion at 12 weeks (Fig. 1C), which is confirmed by CT (Fig. 1D).

Case 2. A 36-year-old female former smoker sustained an open talus fracture-dislocation with associated degloving injury 5 years before presentation. An attempted tibiotalocalcaneal fusion was done with a blade plate. The initial postoperative course was hindered by protracted wound drainage. Most recently she was referred for chronic pain and difficulty with ambulation. The patient's radiographs revealed a varus nonunion (Fig. 2A–C). Because of her history, before conducting a revision preoperative diagnostic studies (indium-111 white blood cell scan, erythrocyte sedimentation rate, c-reactive protein) were acquired. All results were negative

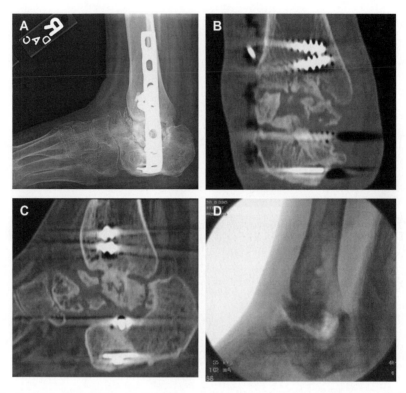

Fig. 2. (*A*) Lateral radiograph displaying nonunion of attempted tibiotalocalcaneal fusion. (*B*) Coronal CT scan image displaying nonunion of attempted tibiotalocalcaneal fusion. (*C*) Sagittal CT scan image displaying nonunion of attempted tibiotalocalcaneal fusion. (*D*) Intra-operative fluoroscopic lateral image demonstrating nonunion after removal of prior hardware. (*E*) Intraoperative fluoroscopic lateral image after fusion surgery done with retrograde nail and BMP 2 augmentation. (*F*) Lateral radiograph 12 weeks after tibiotalocalcaneal fusion surgery demonstrating bony union of fusion sites and alignment restoration. (*G*) Coronal CT scan image 12 weeks after tibiotalocalcaneal fusion surgery demonstrating bony union of fusion sites and alignment restoration. (*H*) Sagittal CT scan image 12 weeks after tibiotalocalcaneal fusion surgery demonstrating bony union of fusion sites and alignment restoration.

for infection. A revision tibiotalocalcaneal fusion was performed with a ret-rograde IMN and adjuvant BMP 2. (Fig. 2D, E) Her postoperative course was uneventful and at 12 weeks she proceeded to union (Fig. 2F–H). At 2-year follow-up she remains pain-free and satisfied with her result [111–118].

Summary

Many reconstructive options exist for symptomatic hindfoot and ankle problems. Hindfoot and tibiotalar fusions are reliable procedures with consistent results. Unfortunately, many potential complications have been cited throughout the literature. Although the most important aspect

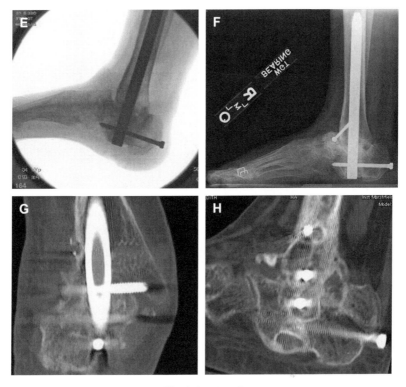

Fig. 2 (*continued*)

in any fusion surgery is meticulous technique, advances in technology, including PRP, bone stimulators, and BMPs seem to be useful additions in the quest to achieve solid fusions with decreased complications.

References

[1] Morrey BF, Wiedeman GP Jr. Complications and long-term results of ankle arthrodesis following trauma. J Bone Joint Surg Am 1980;62(5):777–84.
[2] Frey C, Halikus NM, Vu-Rose T, et al. A review of ankle arthrodesis: predisposing factors to nonunion. Foot Ankle Int 1994;15(11):581–4.
[3] Seitz DG, Carpenter EB. Triple arthrodesis in children: a ten-year review. South Med J 1974;67(12):1420–4.
[4] Haritidis JH, Kirkos JM, Provellegios SM, et al. Long-term results of triple arthrodesis: 42 cases followed for 25 years. Foot Ankle Int 1994;15(10):548–51.
[5] Graves SC, Mann RA, Graves KO. Triple arthrodesis in older adults. Results after long-term follow-up. J Bone Joint Surg Am 1993;75(3):355–62.
[6] Angus PD, Cowell HR. Triple arthrodesis. A critical long-term review. J Bone Joint Surg Br 1986;68(2):260–5.
[7] Kitaoka HB, Patzer GL. Clinical results of the Mayo total ankle arthroplasty. J Bone Joint Surg Am 1996;78(11):1658–64.

[8] Takakura Y, Tanaka Y, Sugimoto K, et al. Ankle arthroplasty. A comparative study of cemented metal and uncemented ceramic prostheses. Clin Orthop Relat Res 1990;(252): 209–16.

[9] Moore TJ, Prince R, Pochatko D, et al. Retrograde intramedullary nailing for ankle arthrodesis. Foot Ankle Int 1995;16(7):433–6.

[10] Dhawan SK, Conti SF, Towers J, et al. The effect of pulsed electromagnetic fields on hindfoot arthrodesis: a prospective study. J Foot Ankle Surg 2004;43(2):93–6.

[11] Saltzman C, Lightfoot A, Amendola A. PEMF as treatment for delayed healing of foot and ankle arthrodesis. Foot Ankle Int 2004;25(11):771–3.

[12] Burkus JK, Transfeldt EE, Kitchel SH, et al. Clinical and radiographic outcomes of anterior lumbar interbody fusion using recombinant human bone morphogenetic protein-2. Spine 2002;27(21):2396–408.

[13] Einhorn TA, Majeska RJ, Mohaideen A, et al. A single percutaneous injection of recombinant human bone morphogenetic protein-2 accelerates fracture repair. J Bone Joint Surg Am 2003;85-A(8):1425–35.

[14] Coetzee JC, Pomeroy GC, Watts JD, et al. The use of autologous concentrated growth factors to promote syndesmosis fusion in the Agility total ankle replacement. A preliminary study. Foot Ankle Int 2005;26(10):840–6.

[15] Bibbo C. Autologous platelet concentrate in high-risk foot & ankle surgery. In: AOFAS 20th Annual Summer Meeting. 07/28–07/31, 2004. Seattle, WA.

[16] Bibbo C, Bono CM, Lin SS. Union rates using autologous platelet concentrate alone and with bone graft in high-risk foot and ankle surgery patients. J Surg Orthop Adv 2005;14(1): 17–22.

[17] el-Batouty MM, Aly ES, el-Lakkany MR, et al. Triple arthrodesis for paralytic valgus– a modified technique: brief report. J Bone Joint Surg Br 1988;70(3):493.

[18] Koenig RJ, Peterson CM, Jones RL, et al. Correlation of glucose regulation and hemoglobin AIc in diabetes mellitus. N Engl J Med 1976;295(8):417–20.

[19] Russotti GM, Cass JR, Johnson KA. Isolated talocalcaneal arthrodesis. A technique using moldable bone graft. J Bone Joint Surg Am 1988;70(10):1472–8.

[20] Sangeorzan BJ, Smith D, Veith R, et al. Triple arthrodesis using internal fixation in treatment of adult foot disorders. Clin Orthop Relat Res 1993;(294):299–307.

[21] Siffert RS, del Torto U. "Beak" triple arthrodesis for severe cavus deformity. Clin Orthop Relat Res 1983;(181):64–7.

[22] Wetmore RS, Drennan JC. Long-term results of triple arthrodesis in Charcot-Marie-Tooth disease. J Bone Joint Surg Am 1989;71(3):417–22.

[23] Bennett GL, Graham CE, Mauldin DM. Triple arthrodesis in adults. Foot Ankle 1991; 12(3):138–43.

[24] Jarde O, Abiraad G, Gabrion A, et al. L'arthrodese medio-tarsienne et soustalienne dans le traitement du pied plat valgus de l'adulte par insuffisance du tendon du tibial posterieur. Resultats d'une serie de 20 cas. Acta Orthop Belg 2002;68(1):56–62.

[25] Mann RA, Rongstad KM. Arthrodesis of the ankle: a critical analysis. Foot Ankle Int 1998;19(1):3–9.

[26] Anderson T, Maxander P, Rydholm U, et al. Ankle arthrodesis by compression screws in rheumatoid arthritis: primary nonunion in 9/35 patients. Acta Orthop 2005;76(6): 884–90.

[27] Chan SC, Alexander IJ. Subtalar arthrodesis with interposition tricortical iliac crest graft for late pain and deformity after calcaneus fracture. Foot Ankle Int 1997;18(10):613–5.

[28] Carreon LY, Glassman SD, Anekstein Y, et al. Platelet gel (AGF) fails to increase fusion rates in instrumented posterolateral fusions. Spine 2005;30(9):E243–6; discussion E247.

[29] Amendola A, Lammens P. Subtalar arthrodesis using interposition iliac crest bone graft after calcaneal fracture. Foot Ankle Int 1996;17(10):608–14.

[30] Weibrich G, Hansen T, Kleis W, et al. Effect of platelet concentration in platelet-rich plasma on peri-implant bone regeneration. Bone 2004;34(4):665–71.

[31] Mangone PG, Fleming LL, Fleming SS, et al. Treatment of acquired adult planovalgus deformities with subtalar fusion. Clin Orthop Relat Res 1997;(341):106–12.

[32] Mann RA, Beaman DN, Horton GA. Isolated subtalar arthrodesis. Foot Ankle Int 1998; 19(8):511–9.

[33] Kitaoka HB, Patzer GL. Subtalar arthrodesis for posterior tibial tendon dysfunction and pes planus. Clin Orthop Relat Res 1997;(345):187–94.

[34] Trnka HJ, Easley ME, Lam PW, et al. Subtalar distraction bone block arthrodesis. J Bone Joint Surg Br 2001;83(6):849–54.

[35] Easley ME, Trnka HJ, Schon LC, et al. Isolated subtalar arthrodesis. J Bone Joint Surg Am 2000;82(5):613–24.

[36] Stuart MJ, Morrey BF. Arthrodesis of the diabetic neuropathic ankle joint. Clin Orthop 1990;(253):209–11.

[37] Papa J, Myerson M, Girard P. Salvage, with arthrodesis, in intractable diabetic neuropathic arthropathy of the foot and ankle. J Bone Joint Surg Am 1993;75(7):1056–66.

[38] Garland DE, Moses B, Salyer W. Long-term follow-up of fracture nonunions treated with PEMFs. Contemp Orthop 1991;22(3):295–302.

[39] Guerkov HH, Lohmann CH, Liu Y, et al. Pulsed electromagnetic fields increase growth factor release by nonunion cells. Clin Orthop Relat Res 2001;(384):265–79.

[40] Spadaro JA, Bergstrom WH. In vivo and in vitro effects of a pulsed electromagnetic field on net calcium flux in rat calvarial bone. Calcif Tissue Int 2002;70(6):496–502.

[41] Bodamyali T, Bhatt B, Hughes FJ, et al. Pulsed electromagnetic fields simultaneously induce osteogenesis and upregulate transcription of bone morphogenetic proteins 2 and 4 in rat osteoblasts in vitro. Biochem Biophys Res Commun 1998;250(2):458–61.

[42] Diniz P, Shomura K, Soejima K, et al. Effects of pulsed electromagnetic field (PEMF) stimulation on bone tissue like formation are dependent on the maturation stages of the osteoblasts. Bioelectromagnetics 2002;23(5):398–405.

[43] Bodamyali T, Kanczler JM, Simon B, et al. Effect of faradic products on direct current-stimulated calvarial organ culture calcium levels. Biochem Biophys Res Commun 1999; 264(3):657–61.

[44] Wang Q, Zhong S, Ouyang J, et al. Osteogenesis of electrically stimulated bone cells mediated in part by calcium ions. Clin Orthop Relat Res 1998;(348):259–68.

[45] Brighton CT, Wang W, Seldes R, et al. Signal transduction in electrically stimulated bone cells. J Bone Joint Surg Am 2001;83-A(10):1514–23.

[46] Zhuang H, Wang W, Seldes RM, et al. Electrical stimulation induces the level of TGF-beta1 mRNA in osteoblastic cells by a mechanism involving calcium/calmodulin pathway. Biochem Biophys Res Commun 1997;237(2):225–9.

[47] Ibiwoye MO, Powell KA, Grabiner MD, et al. Bone mass is preserved in a critical-sized osteotomy by low energy pulsed electromagnetic fields as quantitated by in vivo micro-computed tomography. J Orthop Res 2004;22(5):1086–93.

[48] Inoue N, Ohnishi I, Chen D, et al. Effect of pulsed electromagnetic fields (PEMF) on late-phase osteotomy gap healing in a canine tibial model. J Orthop Res 2002;20(5):1106–14.

[49] Donley BG, Ward DM. Implantable electrical stimulation in high-risk hindfoot fusions. Foot Ankle Int 2002;23(1):13–8.

[50] Lau JS, Myerson M, Schon L. A retrospective analysis of using implantable DC bone stimulators in high risk and revision foot and ankle surgery. Submitted 2005.

[51] Midis N, Conti SF. Revision ankle arthrodesis. Foot Ankle Int 2002;23(3):243–7.

[52] Grotendorst GR, Martin GR, Pencev D, et al. Stimulation of granulation tissue formation by platelet-derived growth factor in normal and diabetic rats. J Clin Invest 1985;76(6): 2323–9.

[53] Joyce ME, Jingushi S, Scully SP, et al. Role of growth factors in fracture healing. Prog Clin Biol Res 1991;365:391–416.

[54] Einhorn TA, Boskey AL, Gundberg CM, et al. The mineral and mechanical properties of bone in chronic experimental diabetes. J Orthop Res 1988;6(3):317–23.

[55] Doxey DL, Ng MC, Dill RE, et al. Platelet-derived growth factor levels in wounds of diabetic rats. Life Sci 1995;57(11):1111–23.

[56] Nash TJ, Howlett CR, Martin C, et al. Effect of platelet-derived growth factor on tibial osteotomies in rabbits. Bone 1994;15(2):203–8.

[57] Fujii H, Kitazawa R, Maeda S, et al. Expression of platelet-derived growth factor proteins and their receptor alpha and beta mRNAs during fracture healing in the normal mouse. Histochem Cell Biol 1999;112(2):131–8.

[58] Thomas T, Gori F, Spelsberg TC, et al. Response of bipotential human marrow stromal cells to insulin-like growth factors: effect on binding protein production, proliferation, and commitment to osteoblasts and adipocytes. Endocrinology 1999;140(11):5036–44.

[59] Canalis E, Rydziel S, Delany AM, et al. Insulin-like growth factors inhibit interstitial collagenase synthesis in bone cell cultures. Endocrinology 1995;136(4):1348–54.

[60] Jonsson KB, Ljunghall S, Karlstrom O, et al. Insulin-like growth factor I enhances the formation of type I collagen in hydrocortisone-treated human osteoblasts. Biosci Rep 1993; 13(5):297–302.

[61] Gangji V, Rydziel S, Gabbitas B, et al. Insulin-like growth factor II promoter expression in cultured rodent osteoblasts and adult rat bone. Endocrinology 1998;139(5): 2287–92.

[62] Mohan S, Baylink DJ. Insulin-like growth factor system components and the coupling of bone formation to resorption. Horm Res 1996;45(Suppl 1):59–62.

[63] Rosen CJ, Donahue LR. Insulin-like growth factors and bone: the osteoporosis connection revisited. Proc Soc Exp Biol Med 1998;219(1):1–7.

[64] Mochizuki H, Hakeda Y, Wakatsuki N, et al. Insulin-like growth factor-I supports formation and activation of osteoclasts. Endocrinology 1992;131(3):1075–80.

[65] Hill PA, Reynolds JJ, Meikle MC. Osteoblasts mediate insulin-like growth factor-I and -II stimulation of osteoclast formation and function. Endocrinology 1995;136(1):124–31.

[66] Canalis E. Insulin like growth factors and the local regulation of bone formation. Bone 1993;14(3):273–6.

[67] Birnbaum RS, Bowsher RR, Wiren KM. Changes in IGF-I and -II expression and secretion during the proliferation and differentiation of normal rat osteoblasts. J Endocrinol 1995; 144(2):251–9.

[68] Andrew JG, Hoyland J, Freemont AJ, et al. Insulinlike growth factor gene expression in human fracture callus. Calcif Tissue Int 1993;53(2):97–102.

[69] Middleton J, Arnott N, Walsh S, et al. Osteoblasts and osteoclasts in adult human osteophyte tissue express the mRNAs for insulin-like growth factors I and II and the type 1 IGF receptor. Bone 1995;16(3):287–93.

[70] Shinar DM, Endo N, Halperin D, et al. Differential expression of insulin-like growth factor-I (IGF-I) and IGF-II messenger ribonucleic acid in growing rat bone. Endocrinology 1993;132(3):1158–67.

[71] Edwall D, Prisell PT, Levinovitz A, et al. Expression of insulin-like growth factor I messenger ribonucleic acid in regenerating bone after fracture: influence of indomethacin. J Bone Miner Res 1992;7(2):207–13.

[72] Robey PG, Young MF, Flanders KC, et al. Osteoblasts synthesize and respond to transforming growth factor-type beta (TGF-beta) in vitro. J Cell Biol 1987;105(1): 457–63.

[73] Sporn MB, Roberts AB. The Multifunctional Nature of Growth Factors. In: Sporn MB, Roberts AB, editors. Handbook of Experimental Pharmacology: Peptide Growth Factors and their Receptors. New York: Springer-Verlag; 1990. p. 3–15.

[74] Canalis E. Effect of growth factors on bone cell replication and differentiation. Clin Orthop Relat Res 1985;193:246–63.

[75] Rickard DJ, Gowen M, MacDonald BR. Proliferative responses to estradiol, IL-1 alpha and TGF beta by cells expressing alkaline phosphatase in human osteoblast-like cell cultures. Calcif Tissue Int 1993;52(3):227–33.

[76] Centrella M, Casinghino S, Ignotz R, et al. Multiple regulatory effects by transforming growth factor-beta on type I collagen levels in osteoblast-enriched cultures from fetal rat bone. Endocrinology 1992;131(6):2863–72.

[77] Wrana JL, Maeno M, Hawrylyshyn B, et al. Differential effects of transforming growth factor-beta on the synthesis of extracellular matrix proteins by normal fetal rat calvarial bone cell populations. J Cell Biol 1988;106(3):915–24.

[78] Joyce ME, Jingushi S, Bolander ME. Transforming growth factor-beta in the regulation of fracture repair. Orthop Clin North Am 1990;21(1):199–209.

[79] Rosen DM, Stempien SA, Thompson AY, et al. Differentiation of rat mesenchymal cells by cartilage-inducing factor. Enhanced phenotypic expression by dihydrocytochalasin B. Exp Cell Res 1986;165(1):127–38.

[80] Seyedin SM, Thomas TC, Thompson AY, et al. Purification and characterization of two cartilage-inducing factors from bovine demineralized bone. Proc Natl Acad Sci U S A 1985;82(8):2267–71.

[81] Babbush CA, Kevy SV, Jacobson MS. An in vitro and in vivo evaluation of autologous platelet concentrate in oral reconstruction. Implant Dent 2003;12(1):24–34.

[82] Kanno T, Takahashi T, Tsujisawa T, et al. Platelet-rich plasma enhances human osteoblast-like cell proliferation and differentiation. J Oral Maxillofac Surg 2005;63(3):362–9.

[83] Gandhi A, Van Gelderen J, Berbarian WS, et al. Platelet releasate enhances healing in patients with a non-union. In: Orthopaedics Research Society 49th Annual Meeting. February 2, 2003. New Orleans, LA.

[84] Barrow CR, Pomeroy GC. Enhancement of syndesmotic fusion rates in total ankle arthroplasty with the use of autologous platelet concentrate. Foot Ankle Int 2005;26(6): 458–61.

[85] Reddi AH. Bone and cartilage differentiation. Curr Opin Genet Dev 1994;4(5):737–44.

[86] Nakajima F, Ogasawara A, Goto K, et al. Spatial and temporal gene expression in chondrogenesis during fracture healing and the effects of basic fibroblast growth factor. J Orthop Res 2001;19(5):935–44.

[87] Bostrom MP, Asnis P. Transforming growth factor beta in fracture repair. Clin Orthop 1998;(355 Suppl):S124–31.

[88] Wozney JM, Rosen V. Bone morphogenetic proteins and their gene expression. In: Noda M, editor. San Diego: Academic Press; 1993. p. 131–67.

[89] Onishi T, Ishidou Y, Nagamine T, et al. Distinct and overlapping patterns of localization of bone morphogenetic protein (BMP) family members and a BMP type II receptor during fracture healing in rats. Bone 1998;22(6):605–12.

[90] Bostrom MP, Lane JM, Berberian WS, et al. Immunolocalization and expression of bone morphogenetic proteins 2 and 4 in fracture healing. J Orthop Res 1995;13(3):357–67.

[91] Ishidou Y, Kitajima I, Obama H, et al. Enhanced expression of type I receptors for bone morphogenetic proteins during bone formation. J Bone Miner Res 1995;10(11):1651–9.

[92] Cho TJ, Gerstenfeld LC, Einhorn TA. Differential temporal expression of members of the transforming growth factor beta superfamily during murine fracture healing. J Bone Miner Res 2002;17(3):513–20.

[93] Lieberman JR, Daluiski A, Einhorn TA. The role of growth factors in the repair of bone. Biology and clinical applications. J Bone Joint Surg Am 2002;84-A(6):1032–44.

[94] Cook SD, Baffes GC, Wolfe MW, et al. The effect of recombinant human osteogenic protein-1 on healing of large segmental bone defects. J Bone Joint Surg Am 1994;76(6): 827–38.

[95] Yasko AW, Lane JM, Fellinger EJ, et al. The healing of segmental bone defects, induced by recombinant human bone morphogenetic protein (rhBMP-2). A radiographic, histological, and biomechanical study in rats. J Bone Joint Surg Am 1992;74(5):659–70.

[96] Bouxsein ML, Turek TJ, Blake CA, et al. Recombinant human bone morphogenetic protein-2 accelerates healing in a rabbit ulnar osteotomy model. J Bone Joint Surg Am 2001; 83-A(8):1219–30.

[97] Govender S, Csimma C, Genant HK, et al. Recombinant human bone morphogenetic protein-2 for treatment of open tibial fractures: a prospective, controlled, randomized study of four hundred and fifty patients. J Bone Joint Surg Am 2002;84-A(12):2123–34.

[98] Johnson EE, Urist MR, Finerman GA. Bone morphogenetic protein augmentation grafting of resistant femoral nonunions. A preliminary report. Clin Orthop Relat Res 1988;(230):257–65.

[99] Friedlaender GE, Perry CR, Cole JD, et al. Osteogenic protein-1 (bone morphogenetic protein-7) in the treatment of tibial nonunions. J Bone Joint Surg Am 2001;83-A(Suppl 1(Pt 2)): S151–8.

[100] Hasharoni A, Zilberman Y, Turgeman G, et al. Murine spinal fusion induced by engineered mesenchymal stem cells that conditionally express bone morphogenetic protein-2. J Neurosurg Spine 2005;3(1):47–52.

[101] Fang J, Zhu YY, Smiley E, et al. Stimulation of new bone formation by direct transfer of osteogenic plasmid genes. Proc Natl Acad Sci U S A 1996;93(12):5753–8.

[102] Chang WH, Chen LT, Sun JS, et al. Effect of pulse-burst electromagnetic field stimulation on osteoblast cell activities. Bioelectromagnetics 2004;25(6):457–65.

[103] Zhu W, Rawlins BA, Boachie-Adjei O, et al. Combined bone morphogenetic protein-2 and -7 gene transfer enhances osteoblastic differentiation and spine fusion in a rodent model. J Bone Miner Res 2004;19(12):2021–32.

[104] Dohm M, Purdy BA, Benjamin J. Primary union of ankle arthrodesis: review of a single institution/multiple surgeon experience. Foot Ankle Int 1994;15(6):293–6.

[105] Crosby LA, Yee TC, Formanek TS, et al. Complications following arthroscopic ankle arthrodesis. Foot Ankle Int 1996;17(6):340–2.

[106] Abdo RV, Wasilewski SA. Ankle arthrodesis: a long-term study. Foot Ankle 1992;13(6): 307–12.

[107] Cracchiolo A 3rd, Cimino WR, Lian G. Arthrodesis of the ankle in patients who have rheumatoid arthritis. J Bone Joint Surg Am 1992;74(6):903–9.

[108] Takakura Y, Tanaka Y, Sugimoto K, et al. Long-term results of arthrodesis for osteoarthritis of the ankle. Clin Orthop Relat Res 1999;(361):178–85.

[109] Ferkel RD, Hewitt M. Long-term results of arthroscopic ankle arthrodesis. Foot Ankle Int 2005;26(4):275–80.

[110] Bednarz PA, Beals TC, Manoli A 2nd. Subtalar distraction bone block fusion: an assessment of outcome. Foot Ankle Int 1997;18(12):785–91.

[111] Sharrard WJ. A double-blind trial of pulsed electromagnetic fields for delayed union of tibial fractures. J Bone Joint Surg Br 1990;72(3):347–55.

[112] Scott G, King JB. A prospective, double-blind trial of electrical capacitive coupling in the treatment of non-union of long bones. J Bone Joint Surg Am 1994;76(6):820–6.

[113] de Haas WG, Beaupre A, Cameron H, et al. The Canadian experience with pulsed magnetic fields in the treatment of ununited tibial fractures. Clin Orthop Relat Res 1986;(208):55–8.

[114] Holmes GB Jr. Treatment of delayed unions and nonunions of the proximal fifth metatarsal with pulsed electromagnetic fields. Foot Ankle Int 1994;15(10):552–6.

[115] Heckman JD, Ingram AJ, Loyd RD, et al. Nonunion treatment with pulsed electromagnetic fields. Clin Orthop Relat Res 1981;(161):58–66.

[116] Paterson DC, Lewis GN, Cass CA. Treatment of delayed union and nonunion with an implanted direct current stimulator. Clin Orthop Relat Res 1980;(148):117–28.

[117] Brighton CT, Pollack SR. Treatment of recalcitrant non-union with a capacitively coupled electrical field. A preliminary report. J Bone Joint Surg Am 1985;67(4):577–85.

[118] Bouillon R, Bex M, Van Herck E, et al. Influence of age, sex, and insulin on osteoblast function: osteoblast dysfunction in diabetes mellitus. J Clin Endocrinol Metab 1995;80(4): 1194–202.

ELSEVIER
SAUNDERS

Foot Ankle Clin N Am
12 (2007) 107–123

FOOT AND
ANKLE CLINICS

Soft Tissue Complications Following Calcaneal Fractures

Troy S. Watson, MD

*Foot and Ankle Institute, Desert Orthopaedic Center, 2800 Desert Inn Road,
Suite 100, Las Vegas, NV 89121, USA*

Since the 1990s, the orthopaedic surgeon's ability to manage calcaneal fractures has improved, increasing the popularity of open reduction and internal fixation. Calcaneal fractures account for most tarsal bone fractures and 2% of all fractures. Clinical studies have examined the effectiveness of operative versus nonoperative treatment of these fractures and the use of computed tomography (CT) has improved the ability to classify a fracture for more accurate comparisons. Howard and colleagues [1] found that significant complications following intra-articular fractures occurred whether treated operatively or nonoperatively and despite management by experienced surgeons. Most of these studies have not focused on soft tissue complications associated with calcaneal fractures. The surgeon's recognition of the various potential soft tissue complications may dampen his enthusiasm to perform operative fixation for these fractures. Soft tissue complications, such as compartment syndrome, fracture blisters, full thickness skin necrosis, and peroneal tendon pathology, can be seen in patients treated nonoperatively, illustrating the point that even conservative management can result in suboptimal outcomes.

The two most feared complications in treating calcaneal fractures with open reduction and internal fixation are wound necrosis and deep infection. Patient selection and timing of the surgical procedure may help reduce the incidence of wound healing problems and infection. When a wound complication occurs, debridement and local wound management play an important initial role. Often these wounds will heal with simple wound care. With the advent of vacuum-assisted wound closure (Wound VAC, KCI, San Antonio, Texas), many of the wounds that would have required a free flap are now being managed with this device. When a wound fails to respond to the above measures, soft tissue coverage is undertaken. Options for coverage

E-mail address: twatson@feetmd.com

range from skin grafts to microsurgical free flaps. Deep infections remain best treated with aggressive debridement and curettage of the bone in conjunction with intravenous antibiotics.

Less common, but potentially equally devastating, is the complication of compartment syndrome of the foot seen in association with calcaneal fractures. Saxby and colleagues [2] found in a series of 98 intra-articular calcaneal fractures that 13% had compartment pressures greater than 30 mm Hg.

Non–limb-threatening complications are also seen as a result of calcaneal fractures. Treatment of these problems is less acute and is typically diagnosed in the later stages of healing. Peroneal tendon tears, impingement, and subluxation have all been reported. Nerve complications, including tarsal tunnel and sural neuromas, have also been seen as sequelae of calcaneal fractures. Even less common, flexor hallucis longus impingement associated with a sustentacular fracture may be seen. Claw toe deformities are occasionally associated with calcaneal fractures, possibly secondary to a missed compartment syndrome of the foot. Often associated with the tongue-type fracture is the development of a Haglund's deformity with associated insertional Achilles tendonitis. The challenge for the surgeon is to recognize the complication and implement the simplest solution to improve the patient's outcome following a calcaneal fracture.

Patient assessment

Many of the wound problems surrounding calcaneal fractures can be attributed to poor decision making at the time of the initial procedure. Special attention to the preoperative assessment of patients before undertaking extensive procedures may lead to a lower incidence of wound complications. Most of this can be completed with a thorough history, a careful extremity exam, and diagnostic testing when necessary.

Medical history

Taking a complete history is important in the surgeon's quest to avoid wound-healing complications. Patients who have diabetes mellitus are at increased risk for the development of postoperative wound complications and infections (Fig. 1). The severity of the complications is not necessarily related to the severity of the disease itself, with type II diabetes accounting for most problems. A careful evaluation of the patient who has diabetes is necessary to document neuropathy, previous foot ulcerations, and adequacy of blood glucose control. A fasting blood glucose and hemoglobin A1c are simple blood tests to obtain and will aid the surgeon in assessing a diabetic patient's compliance and control of his disease. In addition, careful evaluation of the vascular integrity of the limb should be undertaken. Lack of distal pulses warrants further studies, such as arterial Doppler examination with waveforms, ankle-brachial indices, and toe pressures. Suboptimal Doppler results may be a contraindication to surgical management of the

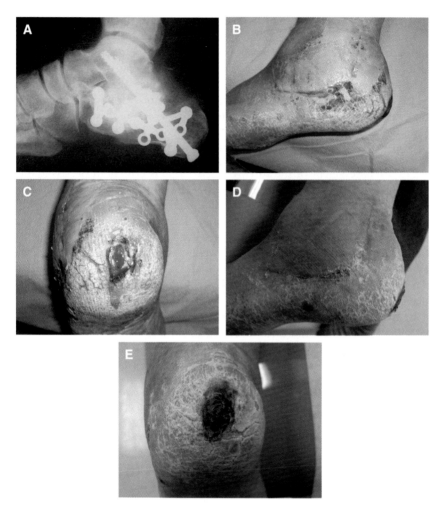

Fig. 1. A patient with type II diabetes presented with a Sander's type IV calcaneal fracture and was treated with open reduction and internal fixation and primary subtalar fusion (*A*). At 1 week from surgical intervention, a wound dehiscence was noted over the lateral wound and posterior heel from screw placement (*B*, *C*). The wounds were debrided in the office and the patient was placed into a removable CAM boot to allow for local care. One week later, wound exam in the office shows improvement in both areas (*D*, *E*).

fracture. Specialists should evaluate all comorbidities, such as renal failure, peripheral vascular disease, and heart disease, before undertaking any surgical procedure.

A careful evaluation of a patient's tobacco use is important in avoiding complications. A history of smoking affects wound healing adversely. Smoking is a relative contraindication to surgical intervention and should be taken into account with all other factors.

Discussing with the patient his social situation and his ability to comply with postoperative instructions can aide in prevention of serious complications. Any underlying psychiatric disorders should be documented. Observation of the patient preoperatively in the office may reveal potential noncompliance issues, which may be amplified once the patient is feeling better. Alcohol and drug abuse that could interfere with postoperative protocols may be a relative contraindication for surgery.

Extremity exam

Careful assessment of the soft tissue envelope is critical in the avoidance of postoperative wounds and infections. The initial surgery should take place only after soft tissue swelling has subsided. The surgical exposure should avoid fracture blisters, especially those filled with blood [3]. Serum-filled blisters are typically unroofed under sterile conditions and allowed to heal while the soft tissue swelling subsides. When the wrinkle test is positive (the skin wrinkles around lateral foot with ankle dorsiflexion indicating adequate reduction in swelling), surgical intervention can be performed safely (Fig. 2A).

In addition, the extremity vascularity should be assessed, with the lack of peripheral pulses leading to a vascular consult. Lymphedema and venous stasis of the extremity may be contraindications to surgery. Neuropathy should also be noted and a discussion with the patient of the potential complications arising from the lack of sensation discussed preoperatively.

Diagnostic testing

In addition to the typical preoperative laboratory values obtained, the surgeon may want to consider other basic indices of nutrition that may indicate poor wound healing potential. The most basic of these include total lymphocyte count ($>1,500/\mu L$), serum albumin (>3.5 g/dL), serum total protein (>6.2 g/dL), hemoglobin (>11 g/dL) and hematocrit ($>32\%$) [4].

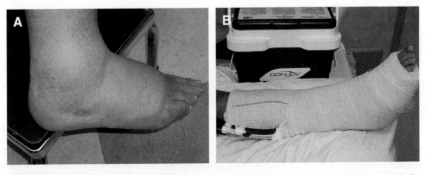

Fig. 2. Closed calcaneal fracture with substantial swelling and failure of the wrinkle test (*A*). Ice therapy and elevation recommended preoperatively to decrease swelling (*B*).

Wound necrosis

The most commonly used approach for operative fixation of calcaneal fractures is the extensile lateral approach popularized by Benirschke and Sangeorzan [5]. In studies reporting wound necrosis complications, the incidence ranges between 2% and 27% [5–9]. The extensile lateral approach was advocated to lessen the number of postoperative wound complications being seen in association with fixation of calcaneal fractures. The lateral flap is supplied entirely by the peroneal artery and its terminal branches. Compromise of this artery from the injury, peripheral vascular disease, and surgical exposure can lead to wound necrosis over the lateral hindfoot. Once a wound develops postoperatively, the surgeon is faced with decisions in the management of the soft tissues. Most of these wounds respond to local wound care modalities, such as debridement and dressing changes. As reported by Folk and colleagues [6] in their series, however, 21% of patients treated operatively required surgical management of their wound complications. Options in the treatment of wound necrosis range from simple wound care to free flaps.

Prevention of wound complications

Many cases of wound necrosis following open reduction and internal fixation of the calcaneus can be avoided with careful surgical planning and patient selection. Often the patient who has a calcaneal fracture presents to the office several days following the initial traumatic event as a referral from the emergency room. Fracture blisters and substantial swelling may be present. Cold therapy and use of a bulky splint are helpful in decreasing swelling and preparing the foot for an operative procedure (Fig. 2B). Use of pneumatic foot pumps can also help decrease swelling if tolerated by the patient. It is not uncommon to wait 1 to 2 weeks for an adequate decrease in swelling as noted with the wrinkle test before safely proceeding with operative fixation. On rare occasion, swelling and blistering may be a relative contraindication to an acute surgical procedure and discussion with the patient of a late reconstruction may be appropriate.

While waiting for subsidence of the swelling, appropriate medical clearance should be obtained. Malnourished patients should undergo laboratory workup with total lymphocyte count, serum albumin, serum protein, hemoglobin, and hematocrit. Patients who have diabetes should undergo a fasting blood glucose and HgA1c level (>8% associated with poor wound healing in diabetic ulcers) [10]. Uncontrolled diabetes should be addressed before surgical intervention. Consultation with an endocrinologist may be helpful in quickly correcting blood glucose levels. Additionally, it should be stressed to the diabetic patient that postoperative tight control of blood glucose levels reduces the rate of wound complications and infections. The lack of palpable pulses is an indication to move forward with an arterial Doppler exam with ankle-brachial indices (ABIs). Patients who have an ABI of <0.8 may have difficulty with wound healing and vascular consult should be obtained with consideration given to nonoperative treatment. Patients who have a history of significant tobacco use or alcohol abuse may not be surgical candidates. Smoking cessation perioperatively may considerably lower the postoperative wound complication rate and patients should be warned of the potential risks of flap necrosis.

Control of intraoperative factors can also reduce the risk for wound healing complications. Extensile exposure allows for some relaxation of the lateral flap with less chance of postoperative breakdown. Use of 0.62-mm Kirschner wires, one placed longitudinally in the fibula and the other placed into the talar neck, may be helpful in providing gentle retraction of the soft tissues. The wires are then bent back providing an excellent retractor of the lateral skin flap (Fig. 3). The surgeon's attention to sharp dissection and avoidance of extensive subcutaneous exploration will lead to fewer soft tissue complications. Care should be taken to avoid injury to the sural nerve and peroneal tendons in the distal portion of the incision.

Once fixation of the calcaneus has been completed, the tourniquet is deflated and hemostasis is obtained. This critical step does take an extra few minutes but can help avoid a postoperative hematoma and its resultant pressure on the lateral skin flap. Occasionally, a small drain can be placed to avoid a hematoma formation although this is not necessary if a dry wound is confirmed after tourniquet release. Nylon suture material is typically preferable to staples. The sutures are placed in a horizontal mattress fashion. The operative foot is then placed into a bulky dressing with a plaster splint and an ice therapy unit, if available, applied.

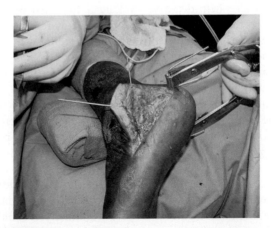

Fig. 3. Extensile lateral approach for ORIF of calcaneal fractures. Note placement of K-wires to allow for gentle retraction of lateral flap.

Treatment of wound complications

Previous studies have illustrated the incidence of wound complications following open reduction and internal fixation to be between 2% and 27%. Once a wound is discovered in the postoperative period there are several measures that can be used in the healing process. Combinations of many of these modalities may be helpful in expediting the healing process and thereby preventing the development of a deep infection. For most postoperative wounds, simple wound care options will likely lead to successful healing.

Local measures

Many of the wounds seen following calcaneal fracture fixation are slight wound dehiscence with minimal drainage. Although the wounds are concerning to the practitioner, most will heal with local measures. Debridement of unhealthy or nonviable tissue remains the most important step in treating all wounds [11]. This procedure is best completed in the office with a #15 scalpel blade and pick-ups with teeth to minimize traumatic injury to the remaining viable soft tissues. A curette can also be an effective tool in the office. Following debridement, wet-to-dry saline dressing changes, when done correctly, are an effective wound healing adjunct. Caustic agents, such as Dakin's solution, should be avoided because they can be irritating to the surrounding soft tissues and lead to a delay in wound closure [12]. With the advent of newer topical debriding preparations containing proteases, papain derivatives, and collagenases, the traditional wet-to-dry dressings are becoming outdated. Preventative oral antibiotics are usually administered to prevent a deep infection and persistent wound healing problems. Dressings should be occlusive in nature while providing for absorption of any exudate.

Vacuum-assisted wound closure

Vacuum-assisted wound closure (VAC) in the treatment of calcaneal wound necrosis has vastly improved the orthopaedic surgeon's ability to manage this complication (Fig. 4). Debridement remains the critical treatment, but the wound VAC can provide substantial assistance. Wounds that formerly would have required a microsurgical free flap are now, in some cases, successfully treated with VAC (Fig. 5) [13].

VAC exposes the wound bed to negative pressure by way of a closed system. Polyurethane foam dressing is placed into the wound and attached to an evacuation tube, which is connected to the vacuum device. The negative pressure created by this system increases tissue perfusion, removes wound debris and fluid, and enhances proliferation of granulation tissue. Cell proliferation is believed to result from a stretching of the cells and cytoskeletal elements. The application of micromechanical forces to a wound may

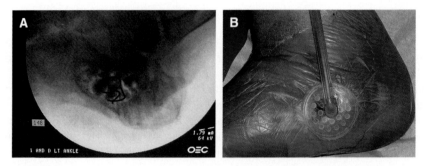

Fig. 4. Wound associated with osteomyelitis of the calcaneus treated with debridement, curettage and placement of antibiotic beads (*A*). VAC was successfully used in conjunction with surgical debridement (*B*).

stimulate healing through promotion of cell proliferation, angiogenesis, and local elaboration of growth factors [14]. In addition to these benefits, VAC may also decrease bacterial cell counts within a wound [15]. This technique can be used in an attempt to close wounds with underlying exposed bone and in some instances exposed hardware (Fig. 6) [16]. In the author's experience, closure of some of these deep wounds in fairly short duration (2 to 6 weeks) has been observed.

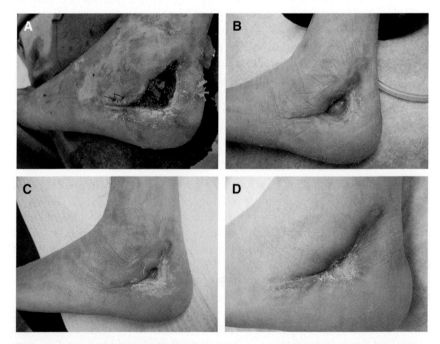

Fig. 5. Lateral wound necrosis noted at two weeks after ORIF of a calcaneal fracture (*A*). Wound treated with debridement in the office and placement of VAC. Four-week (*B*), 6-week (*C*), and 12-week (*D*) follow-up after VAC placement with closure of the wound.

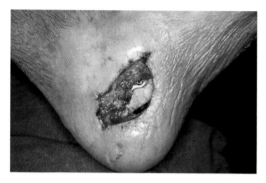

Fig. 6. Lateral wound necrosis with exposed hardware. Successful treatment with VAC eliminated need for pedicle or free flap.

Hyperbaric oxygen

Hyperbaric oxygen (HBO) is currently being used in the treatment of chronic, nonhealing wounds. This typically is not advocated as the sole treatment but rather as an adjunct to other modalities, including local wound care and debridement. Published studies have been criticized for their lack of standardization in data collection making it difficult to interpret the results. Additionally, most studies have a small cohort and lack a comparable control group. One randomized, double-blinded study showed a statistically significant difference in wound size in a group treated with HBO and wound care versus a group that received wound care only. This study only had 16 patients all of whom were nonsmokers and non-diabetics who had normal ABIs, however [17]. Others have found HBO to be ineffective in the treatment of chronic wounds. Ciaravino and colleagues [18] found HBO difficult to justify based on the lack of clinical evidence that it works, its high cost, and potential complications. A meta-analysis on HBO, including randomized and nonrandomized studies, suggests a moderate benefit of the treatment of chronic wounds, although certainly large randomized and controlled studies need to be done to more clearly outline the benefits [19]. The author believes this topic remains a gray area given the conflicting evidence-based research. Use of HBO may serve as a useful adjunct but should not replace traditional proven techniques. Transcutaneous oxygen measurements after an oxygen challenge should increase in those patients who are most likely to benefit from the treatment. Debridement and local wound care remain at the forefront in the treatment of a chronic wound.

Autologous platelet gel

A complex cascade of events that are ultimately modulated by interacting molecular signals, primarily cytokines, and growth factors (GF), mediates wound healing. Several clinical trials have demonstrated that chronic wounds may, in some cases, lack the availability of GF. This lack can be the result of decreased production, decreased release, trapping, excess degradation, or a combination of the above. Deficiencies of GF in chronic wounds suggest a role for therapeutic use to accelerate the tissue-healing process. Several studies have documented the efficacy of topical GF management on animal models and human subjects with promising results [20–22].

Platelets play a critical role in wound healing. During the coagulation and inflammation phases of healing, the formation of a blood clot induces adhesion, aggregation, and degranulation of circulating platelets. Platelet alpha granules release numerous growth factors important to tissue remodeling [20]. Autogenous platelet gel is created by treating platelet concentrates with autologous thrombin obtained by differential centrifugation of whole blood. This gel is then applied to the wound with an occlusive dressing. Further clinical trials will need to be done to elucidate the efficacy of this treatment of chronic foot and ankle wounds.

Coverage for larger wounds

In rare cases, the postoperative wound complication around a calcaneal fracture may require more substantial measures to close the wound. Options for closure of these difficult wounds include skin grafts, local flaps, pedicle flaps, and microsurgical free flaps.

Skin grafting requires a clean, well-vascularized base. A skin graft will typically not take if there is underlying infection or fibrous tissue present. VAC is an excellent technique to prepare the wound for skin grafting because it promotes granulation tissue and decreases bacterial cell counts. In fact, VAC can be used over a skin graft to promote take of the graft. Application of a nonadherent dressing with a bolster, topical antibiotics, and a compressive dressing can be helpful in increasing the rate of take of the graft.

Local flaps are flaps whose success depends on a length-to-width ratio (1:1) with no specific blood flow at their base. An example of such a flap is a rotation flap. These flaps are typically not useful in lateral hindfoot wounds because there is little skin redundancy for skin coverage, and they are therefore not recommended [13].

In contrast to local flaps, the pedicled flaps have a defined blood supply at their base. This type of flap brings in vascularized tissue that can cover exposed bone and hardware. Wounds that are smaller than 4 to 5 cm^2 can be considered for a pedicled flap. These flaps are typically easy to harvest, provide a vascularized coverage of the exposed area, and the donor site can be closed primarily. The disadvantages of these flaps are their limited bulk and reach [23]. The main workhorse for lateral hindfoot and distal ankle wounds is the abductor digiti minimi muscle flap, which is supplied by the lateral plantar artery. The donor site can be primarily closed following harvest [13]. One other flap that is commonly used for lateral ankle and

hindfoot defects is the sural artery flap. This flap is capable of covering defects up to 10 cm × 13 cm [24]. This flap provides for primary closure of the
donor site but has disadvantages, including venous congestion and a complication rate of up to 25% in high-risk patients [25].

Microsurgical free flaps provide certain advantages over those flaps discussed above. These flaps can cover large defects and improve perfusion
of infected bone. The disadvantages include longer operating times, increased perioperative complications, and technical difficulty. Microsurgical
technique allows the surgeon to obtain healthy tissue from a distant site
and transfer it to the lateral calcaneus area where the vascular pedicle is
anastomosed to the local existing blood supply.

Open calcaneal fracture management

There currently is no widely accepted protocol in the treatment of open
calcaneal fractures. These tend to be high-energy fractures and the initial in-
sult to the soft tissues is significant resulting in a higher incidence of postoperative complications. Although much has been written on the treatment of
other open fractures, little has been written about the management of open
calcaneal fractures [9,26–29]. The reason for the paucity of literature is likely
because of the low frequency of these fractures. Over a 9-year period, Heier
and associates [27] treated 43 open calcaneal fractures and 503 closed fractures. Open calcaneal fractures thus represented only 7.9% of all calcaneal
fractures in their institution.

Most investigators concur that management of the soft tissues and intravenous (IV) antibiotics compose the initial phase of treatment. Surgical irrigation and debridement (I & D) urgently from the emergency room and
every 24 to 48 hours thereafter until the wound is clean typically is recommended. There is great controversy over placement of hardware, internal
fixation versus percutaneous pin fixation, and the timing of such a procedure. Even with appropriate wound management, patients should be ap-
prised of the possibility of a soft tissue complication. Thorton and
colleagues [29], in an attempt to answer some of these questions, designed
a treatment protocol algorithm for open calcaneal fractures. Initial management involved I & D of the traumatic wound until clean. They concluded
that calcaneal fractures with any size lateral wound, a medial wound greater
than 4 cm, a wound that cannot be closed, and an unstable wound at 7 to 10
days following the injury should be treated with open reduction and percutaneous stabilization. In patients who have a medial wound less than 4 cm
that has been closed and stable for 7 to 10 days, standard techniques for
open reduction and internal fixation can be used. Complication rates using
this protocol were 29% (9/31). Future studies in this area should examine
other algorithms and consideration should be given to initial soft tissue
management followed by late reconstruction.

Compartment syndrome of the foot

Little has been written about compartment syndromes associated with calcaneal fractures. In fact, controversy surrounds whether or not this represents a clinically significant entity in the face of a calcaneal fracture and what, if any, treatment is necessary. Clinical suspicion arises based on examination that shows pain out of proportion to what is typically seen with a calcaneal fracture and tense swelling of the foot. Compartment pressures are then obtained with multistick invasive catheterization, especially of the calcaneal compartment of the hindfoot. Approximately 10% of calcaneal fractures develop compartment syndromes of the foot. Previous reports commented on the need for immediate fasciotomy to prevent the development of ischemic contractures [30]. More recently, however, Myerson and colleagues [31] concluded that the use of intermittent compression foot pumps decreases elevated compartment pressures associated with calcaneal fractures and may obviate the need for acute fasciotomies. Late reconstruction can then be performed, if necessary. Sequelae of compartment syndromes of the foot can include chronic neurogenic pain and neurovascular compromise leading to sensory disturbances in the medial or lateral plantar nerve distribution and ischemic contractures, including claw toe deformities (Fig. 7). Early treatment of the claw toe deformities may include a simple toe flexor tenotomy to prevent further deformity. Late treatment is best provided with proximal interphalangeal joint resection and pinning or flexor to extensor transfer if the deformity is flexible.

Neuritis

Nerve problems, including neuromas and compression syndromes, can be seen as late sequelae in the treatment of calcaneal fractures. Most commonly this is in the form of a sural neuritis/neuroma or tarsal tunnel syndrome.

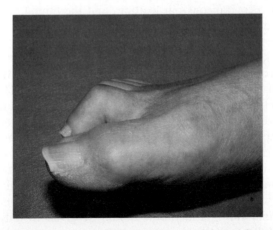

Fig. 7. Claw toe deformities seen following a calcaneal fracture.

The extensile approach allows for identification of the sural nerve proximally and occasionally distally. This approach usually results in avoidance of nerve injury to the sural nerve. Nonetheless, sural nerve injuries do occur, possibly from retraction, contusion from the original injury, or cut by the surgeon. Diagnosis is mainly clinical and a differential injection with steroid may be trialed to alleviate symptoms. Often, surgical intervention is necessary to excise the painful neuroma. The site of the neuroma is marked before surgery. Dissection should identify the neuroma, which is then transected. The remaining nerve is then carefully dissected from the soft tissue scar and traced proximally into the distal ankle region where it can be buried in the peroneal brevis muscle belly without tension.

Tarsal tunnel syndrome after calcaneal fractures can be seen as a result of scarring or heel widening secondary to the original fracture [32,33]. Tarsal tunnel release is indicated if compression of the tibial nerve is noted by clinical exam. The author prefers to have supporting neurodiagnostic evidence of tarsal tunnel syndrome before proceeding with release of the tarsal tunnel. The surgeon should delay surgery several months following the index procedure allowing for all swelling to subside and potential nerve contusions to recover before surgical intervention.

Tendon pathology

In the evaluation of the patient following a calcaneal fracture, persistent pain over the lateral hindfoot could be secondary to painful retained hardware, sural nerve pathology, arthritis of the subtalar or calcaneocuboid joint, or peroneal tendon pathology. To differentiate the potential sources of pain, differential injections can be used. Subtalar joint injections are relatively easy to do in the office without the need for fluoroscopic guidance. If the calcaneocuboid joint is suspected as being the pain generator, use of fluoroscopy will ensure correct placement of the injection. Finally, the peroneal tendon sheath and sural nerve can be injected to differentiate these areas. Myerson and Quill [34] found these blocks were helpful in 87.5% of their patients in determining the underlying cause of pain.

The peroneal tendons should be palpated along their course. Resisted eversion may aggravate symptoms and testing for peroneal subluxation can detect this entity. Often, subclinical peroneal tendon subluxation goes undetected with the focus being treatment of the calcaneal fracture. Additionally, especially in the calcaneal fracture treated nonoperatively, calcaneofibular abutment may lead to impingement of the peroneal tendons and chronic pain. CT can sometimes aid the practitioner by identifying subfibular impingement and allowing examination of the integrity of the subtalar and calcaneocuboid joints (Fig. 8A).

Treatment of peroneal tendon tears involves either tubularization (if <50% of the tendon is involved) or tenodesis to the neighboring tendon

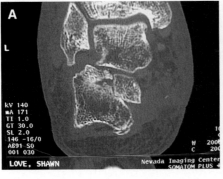
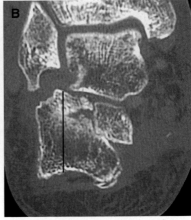

Fig. 8. Patient presented with a grade II open calcaneal fracture with substantial swelling and questionable infection over medial wound. Treated with irrigation and debridement, IV antibiotics, and elevation. Nonoperative management chosen for treatment of the fracture because swelling remained significant at 6 weeks. Patient later presented with subfibular impingement of the peroneal tendons and subtalar joint arthritis (A). Lateral calcaneal wall decompression and subtalar fusion performed as delayed reconstruction (B).

(if > 50% of the tendon is involved) (Fig. 9) [35]. Often lateral calcaneal wall decompression is necessary at the time of peroneal tendon repair as determined by the CT scan. This decompression is accomplished with a wide osteotome and mallet. Care should be taken to ensure adequate bony decompression so that the lateral calcaneal wall no longer abuts the distal fibula (Fig. 8B). In addition, as indicated by Myerson and Quill [34], attention to the subtalar joint is necessary to avoid later need for subtalar fusion. If peroneal tendon dislocation is noted, a fibular groove-deepening procedure with reefing of the superior extensor retinaculum may be indicated. Other procedures, such as those discussed by Chrisman and Snook [36] and

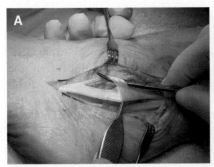
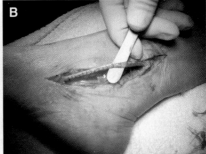

Fig. 9. Peroneal tendon tears may be associated with calcaneal fractures (A). Tubularization is preferred for tears that represent less than 50% of the tendon (B).

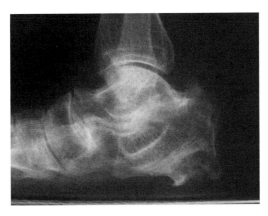

Fig. 10. Haglund's deformity with secondary pain at the insertion of the Achilles tendon was seen in this patient with an old, well-healed, tongue-type fracture of the calcaneus. Also note significant subtalar joint arthrosis.

modified by Acevedo and Myerson [37], can also be helpful in the patient with dislocating peroneal tendons.

Flexor hallucis longus (FHL) tendon scarring, tears, and impingement can also be seen over the medial hindfoot, especially in cases that involve a sustentacular tali fracture. CT scan should rule out a nonunion of this fracture as the cause of pain and may show exostosis impinging the FHL tendon. This rare late sequelae is best treated by exostectomy and tenosynovectomy or repair of the FHL as needed.

Tongue-type fractures displaced by the unopposed pull of the Achilles tendon can be the cause of soft tissue embarrassment and require urgent reduction and fixation. Because of the tenuous soft tissue coverage posterior to the tuberosity of the calcaneus, this type of fracture may tent the skin requiring emergent reduction to avoid disastrous wound complications. The late complications of nonunion and malunion, or perhaps those treated successfully with open reduction and internal fixation, are insertional Achilles tendonitis and Haglund's deformity (Fig. 10). This complication is best diagnosed by physical exam and a weight-bearing lateral radiograph of the foot. Treatment consists of hardware removal if present and a decompression of the Achilles tendon. Haglund's resection and distal reattachment of the Achilles tendon with bioabsorbable suture anchors can resolve symptoms. Care is taken to keep some distal fibers of the Achilles tendon attached to bone while performing the ostectomy of the calcaneus. Equinus contractures should be addressed through a gastrocnemius recession.

Summary

Soft tissue complications following calcaneal fractures can be frustrating to the patient and present reconstructive challenges for the surgeon.

Preoperative patient assessment may define a group of patients who are best treated nonoperatively in an effort to avoid disastrous soft tissue complications. Late sequelae will continue to be seen and through the use of differential injections, physical exam, and appropriate intervention the practitioner can usually decrease symptoms and improve a patient's function. Further studies in the treatment of open calcaneal fractures are necessary to better define treatment algorithms. A working knowledge of these complications and their management is necessary for the surgeon treating calcaneal fractures.

References

[1] Howard JL, Buckley R, McCormack R, et al. Complications following management of displaced intra-articular calcaneal fractures: a prospective randomized trial comparing open reduction internal fixation with nonoperative management. J Orthop Trauma 2003;17(4): 241–9.

[2] Saxby T, Myerson M, Schon L. Compartment syndrome of the foot following calcaneus fracture. Foot 1992;2:157.

[3] Giordano CP, Koval KJ. Treatment of fracture blisters: a prospective study of 53 cases. J Orthop Trauma 1995;9(2):171–6.

[4] Dickhaut S, DeLee J, Page C. Nutritional status: importance in predicting wound-healing after amputation. J Bone Joint Surg Am 1984;66:71–5.

[5] Benirschke SK, Sangeorzan BJ. Extensive intra-articular fractures of the foot: surgical management of calcaneal fractures. Clin Orthop 1993;291:128–34.

[6] Folk JW, Starr AJ, Early JS. Early wound complications of operative treatment of calcaneal fractures: analysis of 190 fractures. J Orthop Trauma 1999;13(5):369–72.

[7] Stephenson JR. Surgical treatment of displaced intraarticular fractures of the calcaneus, a combined medial and lateral approach. Clin Othop 1993;290:68–75.

[8] Abidi NA, Dhawan S, Gruen G, et al. Wound healing risk factors after open reduction and internal fixation of calcaneal fractures. Foot Ankle Int 1999;19:856–61.

[9] Benirschke SK, Kramer PA. Wound healing complications in closed and open calcaneal fractures. J Orthop Trauma 2004;18(1):1–6.

[10] Mantey I, Foster AV, Spencer S, et al. Why do ulcers recur in diabetic foot wounds? Diabet Med 1999;16(3):245–9.

[11] Attinger CE, Bulan EJ. Debridement—the key initial step in wound healing. Foot Ankle Clin 2001;6(4):627–60.

[12] Younger A, Goetz T. Soft tissue coverage for posttraumatic reconstruction. Foot Ankle Clin 2006;11(1):217–35.

[13] Attinger C, Cooper P. Soft tissue reconstruction for calcaneal fractures or osteomyelitis. Orthop Clin North Am 2001;32(1):135–70.

[14] Saxena SM, Hwang CW, Huang S, et al. Vacuum-assisted closure: microdeformations of the wound and cell proliferation. Plast Reconstr Surg 2004;114:1086–96.

[15] Morykwas MJ, Argenta LC, Shelton-Brown EI, et al. Vacuum-assisted closure: a new method for wound control and treatment: animal studies and basic foundation. Ann Plast Surg 1997;38:553–62.

[16] Webb LX. New techniques in wound management: vacuum-assisted wound closure. J Am Acad Orthop Surg 2002;10:303–11.

[17] Hammarlund C, Sundberg T. Hyperbaric oxygen reduced the size of chronic leg ulcers: a randomized double-blind study. Plast Reconstr Surg 1994;93:829–34.

[18] Ciaravino ME, Friedell ML, Kammerlocher TC. Is hyperbaric oxygen a useful adjunct in the management of problem lower extremity wounds? Ann Vasc Surg 1996;10(6):558–62.

[19] Roeckl-Wieddmann I, Bennett M, Kranke P, et al. Systematic review of hyperbaric oxygen in the management of chronic wounds. British J Surg 2005;92:24–32.

[20] Crovetti G, Martinelli G, Issi M, et al. Platelet gel for healing cutaneous chronic wounds. Transfus Apher Sci 2004;30(2):145–51.

[21] Mazzucco L, Medici D, Serra M, et al. The use of platelet gel to treat difficult-to-heal wounds: a pilot study. Transfusion 2004;44:1013–8.

[22] Xia YP, Zhao Y, Marcus J, et al. Effects of keratinocyte growth factor on wound healing in a ischaemic-impaired rabbit ear model and on scar formation. J Pathol 1999;188:431–8.

[23] Attinger CE, Ducic I, Cooper P, et al. The role of intrinsic muscle flaps of the foot for bone coverage in foot and ankle defects in diabetic and nondiabetic patients. Plast Reconstr Surg 2002;110(4):1047–54.

[24] Masquelet AC, Romana MC, Wolf G. Skin island flaps supplied by the vascular axis of the sensitive superficial nerves: anatomic study and clinical experience in the leg. Plast Reconstr Surg 1992;89:1115–21.

[25] Baumeister S, Germann G. Soft tissue coverage of the extremely traumatized foot and ankle. Foot Ankle Clin 2001;6:867–903.

[26] Siebert CH, Hansen M, Wolter D. Follow-up evaluation of open intra-articular fractures of the calcaneus. Arch Orthop Trauma Surg 1998;117(8):442–7.

[27] Heier KA, Infante AF, Walling AK, et al. Open fractures of the calcaneus: soft tissue injury determines outcome. J Bone Joint Surg Am 2003;85(12):2276–82.

[28] Aldridge JM III, Easley M, Nunley JA. Open calcaneal fractures. J Orthop Trauma 2004; 18(1):7–11.

[29] Thorton SJ, Cheleuitte D, Ptaszek AJ, et al. Treatment of open intra-articular calcaneal fractures: evaluation of a treatment protocol based on wound location and size. Foot Ankle Int 2006;27(5):317–23.

[30] Myerson M, Manoli A. Compartment syndromes of the foot after calcaneal fractures. Clin Orthop Relat Res 1993;290:142–50.

[31] Myerson MS, Juliano PJ, Koman JD. The use of pneumatic intermittent impulse compression device in the treatment of calcaneus fractures. Mil Med 2000;165(10):721–5.

[32] Edwards EG, Lincoln CR, Bassett FH III, et al. The tarsal tunnel syndrome: diagnosis and treatment. JAMA 1969;207:716–20.

[33] Byank RP, Clark HJ, Bleeker ML. Standardized neurometric evaluation in tarsal tunnel syndrome. Adv Orthop Surg 1989;12:249.

[34] Myerson MS, Quill GE Jr. Late complications of fractures of the calcaneus. J Bone Joint Surg Am 1993;75:331–41.

[35] Krause JO, Brodsky JW. Peroneus brevis tendon tears: pathophysiology, surgical reconstruction, and clinical results. Foot Ankle Int 1998;19(5):271–9.

[36] Chrisman OD, Snook GA. Reconstruction of lateral ligament tears of the ankle: an experimental study and clinical evaluation of seven patients treated by a new modification of the Elmslie procedure. J Bone Joint Surg Am 1969;51:904–12.

[37] Acevedo JI, Myerson MS. Modification of the Chrisman-Snook technique. Foot Ankle Int 2000;21(2):154–5.

ELSEVIER
SAUNDERS

Foot Ankle Clin N Am
12 (2007) 125–135

FOOT AND
ANKLE CLINICS

Calcaneus Malunion and Nonunion

Verrabdhadra Reddy, MD[a],*, Tomiko Fukuda, MD[a],
Amy Jo Ptaszek, MD[b]

[a]Department of Orthopedic Surgery, Northwestern University Memorial Hospital,
Northwestern University, 645 N. Michigan Avenue, Suite 910, Chicago, IL 60611, USA
[b]Northwestern University Medical School, Illinois Bone and Joint Institute, Ltd.,
2401 Ravine Way, Glenview, IL 60025, USA

Calcaneal fractures have received much attention in the literature over the past century. In part, this attention is due to the fact that it is the most frequently fractured tarsal bone comprising 65% of tarsal injuries [1]. Additionally, the impact of these fractures is increased because they most commonly occur in a young, working subset of the population, resulting in a large economic impact [2]. Thus, many authors have devised different treatment algorithms for calcaneus fractures with little consensus beyond the debilitating deformity that results from the fracture.

Historically authors favored the delayed treatment of calcaneus fractures because of the difficulty of acute fracture treatment and associated complications. In 1908, Cotton [3] described the closed reduction of calcaneus fractures, but eventually transitioned to delayed treatment of the malunion. In 1935, Conn [4] described the traumatic flatfoot with its associated pathology and championed the triple or double arthrodesis to correct the deformity. Gallie [5] followed this in 1943 with the belief that fusion of the midfoot resulted in significant disability and should be restricted to subtalar arthrodesis. Recently, the orthopedic community has become more aggressive with the treatment of calcaneus fractures. The basic principles of articular fracture fixation and the continued evolution of technology have fueled this revival of acute operative intervention. It is also the understanding of the significant deformity and disability associated with conservative management of acute fractures and the resulting malunions or nonunions that have driven the search for a better solution.

* Corresponding author.
E-mail address: vkr593@md.northwestern.edu (V. Reddy).

1083-7515/07/$ - see front matter © 2007 Elsevier Inc. All rights reserved.
doi:10.1016/j.fcl.2006.12.004

foot.theclinics.com

Anatomy

The normal anatomy of the calcaneus is well defined. It is the posterior base of the foot dictating the alignment of the hindfoot and the length of the lateral column. The articular surface is composed of three facets—the posterior, middle, and anterior facets—that are primarily responsible for inversion and eversion of the subtalar joint. The posterior facet is the largest of the three with a convex articulating surface, which is the primary load-bearing surface of the subtalar joint [6]. The middle and anterior facets are separated from the posterior facet by the calcaneal sulcus [7]. The middle facet sits above the sustentaculum with the anterior facet just anterior and lateral to it. The sustentaculum tali arises anterior medially from the body of the calcaneus and supports the talar neck through the anterior and middle facets [7]. The lateral wall of the calcaneus is a relatively thin, flat structure with the peroneal tubercle guiding the peroneal tendons within their respective grooves. The posterior tuberosity is the insertion point of the achilles tendon with its base forming the primary weight bearing structure of the hindfoot [6].

The internal architecture of the calcaneus is such that it is perfect for its primary function of transmitting forces through the posterior and anterior facets. A dense network of longitudinal trabeculae joins with the transverse trabeculae to support the articular facets [8]. The lower pole of the posterior tuberosity, the upper surface at the angle of Gissane and the lateral surface below the anterior portion of the posterior facet have the thickest cortical surfaces in the calcaneus [8]. This framework however creates the neutral triangle as described by Wood [9] and Harty [7], which is composed of very sparse trabecular bone inferior to the lateral process of the talus.

Two angles of reference used to define the normal form of the calcaneus are the crucial angles of Gissane and Bohler's angle. The angle of Gissane is formed by convergence of dense cortical bone from the lateral aspect of the posterior facet with the lateral aspect of the anterior beak of the calcaneus. The normal angle is approximately 90 to 105 degrees [10]. The tuber angle of Bohler [11] is measured between a line extending from the anterior process to the highest point of the posterior facet and another line extending from this point to the superior point of the tuberosity, with normal defined as 20 to 40 degrees. These two reference angles allow a point of comparison when interpreting radiographs of the calcaneus.

Anatomy of the fracture

Calcaneal fractures are most commonly secondary to high-energy trauma such as a fall from a height or a motor vehicle accident [10,11]. The force transferred through the subtalar joint drives the lateral process of the talus into the everted calcaneus to create the fracture patterns described by Essex-Lopresti [10]. The primary fracture line is created by the impaction of the lateral process of the talus into lateral wall of the calcaneus and extends posteromedially into the sustentaculum and the medial wall, producing a fracture line that runs superior lateral to inferior medial [10]. The sustentaculum and medial fragment are held in place relative to the talus by strong talocalcaneal ligaments [12]. The force can then exit anteriorly into the calcaneocuboid joint or the anterior facet. This creates the lateral tuberosity fragment and the medial sustentacular piece [10–12]. The secondary fracture line results from a continuation of the impaction of the talus into the calcaneus. As described by Essex-Lopresti [10], the secondary fracture begins at the apex of the angle of Gissane and exits superiorly just posterior to the posterior facet to produce a joint depression pattern, or it exits inferiorly through the tuberosity to produce a tongue-type fracture.

Carr and colleagues [15] created a cadaveric model of the calcaneal fracture that confirmed the pattern described by Essex-Lopresti. Sabry and colleagues [8] demonstrated the neutral triangle is an area of sparse (60%) or absent (40%) trabeculae just inferior to the lateral process of the talus. This further establishes the mechanism postulated by Essex-Lopresti as the lateral process acts as a wedge driving into this weak region of the calcaneus to create the primary and secondary fracture lines. The resulting fracture pattern leads to the basis of the malunited calcaneus fracture if managed nonoperatively.

Anatomy of the malunion

Understanding the radiographic and anatomic basis of calcaneal fractures is critical to understanding the deformity that will result from conservative treatment of displaced fractures. The displacement of the articular surface of the posterior facet by greater than 2 mm has a significant effect upon its load-bearing characteristics and is known to be a direct cause of arthrosis of the subtalar joint [13–15]. As a result of the fracture, the tuberosity fragment described by Essex-Lopresti translates laterally and superiorly in relation to the sustentaculum effectively decreasing the height of the calcaneus while increasing its width [10–12]. The increased width, or lateral wall exostosis, is a pathologic deformity because it is a direct cause of both subfibular impingement and peroneal tendinopathy or displacement [16–18]. The decreased height of the calcaneus has significant ramifications because it alters the lever arm function of the calcaneus and flattens both the talar inclination and the talocalcaneal angle [19,20]. The loss of the talocalcaneal angle leads to tibiotalar impingement and loss of dorsiflexion [19]. The ultimate constellation of symptoms that patients present with will be dependant on the combination of increased heel width, decreased calcaneal height, and hindfoot varus (Figs. 1 and 2).

Radiographic evaluation

Radiographic evaluation of the malunion differs little from that of the evaluation of acute calcaneus fractures. Standard plain roentgenographic

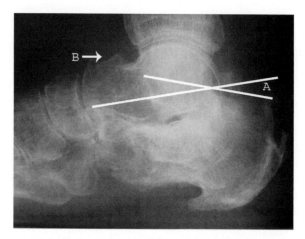

Fig. 1. (*A*) Decrease in Bohler's Angle. (*B*) Anterior osteophyte indicative of tibiotalar impingement.

anteroposterior, lateral, and axial views are a good starting point. The lateral view is used to determine Bohler's angle, talocalcaneal angle, talar declination angle, and height of the calcaneus. Bohler's angle is an indication to the level of depression of the posterior facet or flattening of the calcaneus. A line representing the central axis of the calcaneus and its intersection with a similar line drawn through the talus measures the talocalcaneal angle [19,20]. Talar declination is determined by the angle of the talar axis relative to the plane of support [19]. Both the talar declination angle and the talocalcaneal angle decrease with increasing deformity of the calcaneus and indicate tibiotalar impingement [19,20]. This can become apparent on the lateral view as talar neck erosion. The axial Harris view is used to assess

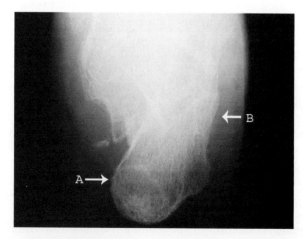

Fig. 2. (*A*) Varus malunion on axial Harris view. (*B*) Lateral wall exostosis.

relative varus/valgus position of the calcaneus and can also appreciate widening of the calcaneus. Broden's [21] view of the posterior facet is used to determine the amount of displacement and evaluate the subtalar joint. The anterior-posterior and lateral views can also be used to evaluate the calcaneocuboid and talonavicular joints for arthrosis.

The evolution of radiographic technology made the computed tomography scan the most reliable and useful tool for evaluating calcaneal malunions. Crosby and Fitzgibbons [22] used the computed tomography scan to assess the amount of displacement of the posterior facet and its prognostic value for closed management of calcaneal fractures. Type I fractures have less than 2 mm of diastases or depression of the fragments. Type II fractures have greater than 2 mm of diastases or depression of the fragments. Type III fractures have severe comminution of the posterior facet. In their series of 13 type I fractures, there were no poor results, but 7 of 7 type III fractures had poor results with closed treatment. There was no correlation between a decrease in Bohler's or Gissane's angle and the final result, but a direct correlation between outcome and the level of comminution of the posterior facet [22]. Stephens and Sanders [23] used coronal images at the level of the posterior facet to create a classification system for calcaneal malunions. Type I malunions have a large lateral wall exostosis without any involvement of the subtalar joint. Type II malunions demonstrate a large lateral wall exostosis and arthrosis of the subtalar joint. Finally, type III malunions have a large lateral wall exostosis, arthrosis of the subtalar joint, and greater than 10 degrees of hindfoot varus. In the initial study of 26 malunions, treatments were rendered according to the type of malunion resulting in significant clinical improvement even with the worst of malunions.

Clinical evaluation

A patient's clinical presentation can aid in isolating the specific issues that need to be addressed. Many patients will complain of difficulty with shoe wear due to the increased width of the hindfoot and difficulty walking on uneven ground secondary to subtalar arthrosis [16–18,24]. Patients may complain of pain at the lateral aspect of the hindfoot that can be due to subfibular impingement, peroneal tendonitis, or subluxation of the tendons. At times it can be difficult to distinguish this pain from subtalar arthrosis [16,17]. An injection of lidocaine into the subtalar joint may help differentiate the source of pain and radiographic correlation may aid in the diagnosis [17]. Evaluation of the patients gait and position of the hindfoot is also important. Collapse of the hindfoot into varus or valgus can cause significant deforming forces on the midfoot and forefoot resulting in an abnormal gait [24]. Patients may also complain of difficulty dorsiflexing the ankle because of tibiotalar impingement [19,25]. Physical examination will demonstrate decreased dorsiflexion of the ankle compared with the contra lateral ankle.

Surgical correction of calcaneal malunions

The significant effect that calcaneal malunions have upon this generally young active population has lead many authors to propose different solutions to create a painless plantigrade foot. Cotton [3] described the correction of the calcaneal malunion by lateral wall exostectomy, correction of hindfoot malalignment, and manipulation of the subtalar joint. Kalamachi and Evans used subtalar arthrodesis technique as described by Gallie [5] and lateral wall exostectomy as described by Conn [4] for treatment of the subtalar arthrosis and lateral wall impingement [26].

Braly and colleagues [17] felt that a significant amount of pain was from the lateral wall exostosis and peroneal tendon pathology. They performed a lateral wall exostectomy for subfibular impingement and/or addressed peroneal pathology, such as tendinopathy, dislocation, or stenosis. One group had prior subtalar fusions but continued to have lateral ankle pain. Six of 8 patients had satisfactory results after lateral exostosis and treatment of peroneal pathology. Group II underwent lateral wall decompression instead of subtalar arthrodesis for treatment of the pain, and 9 of 11 patients had satisfactory outcomes. This points to the importance of being able to isolate the cause of the patient's pain, which can be multifactor in a calcaneal malunion [17].

Carr and colleagues [19] described a subtalar bone block arthrodesis with lateral wall decompression to eliminate the subtalar joint pain, lateral impingement, and tibiotalar impingement. The use of a medial femoral distractor with a tricortical iliac crest autograft allows the correction of the varus collapse, and the distraction of the subtalar joint recreates the talocalcaneal angle. At 1 year, 6 out of 8 patients had satisfactory results, but there was one nonunion, and 2 patients had varus malunions that required reoperation. Bednarz and colleagues [27] performed a subtalar bone block arthrodesis on 29 feet in 28 patients and had a statistically significant improvement in American Orthopaedic Foot and Ankle Society Ankle-Hindfoot score from 25 to 75 ($P < .0001$), and all but 1 patient was satisfied with the outcome (96%). They did have four nonunions and two varus malunions. Of note, the four nonunions only occurred in smokers (4/14 patients). Burton and colleagues [25] had 11 of 13 feet with very satisfactory or satisfactory outcomes using the same protocol and did not have any nonunions or varus malunions at an average follow up of 47 months (25–75 months).

Romash [28] described a technique for correction of the calcaneal malunion by reversing the deformity caused by the original fracture. The osteotomy recreates the superolateral to inferomedial and anterolateral to posteromedial fracture line to produce the sustentacular and tuberosity fragments. The oblique plain is then used to translate the tuberosity fragment inferiorly and medially and then fuse the subtalar joint. This effectively addresses all deformities of the malunion as it increases the calcaneal height while decreasing its width and correcting the varus deformity. In his series of 10 patients with an average follow up of 14 months, 9 had satisfactory results with no reported nonunion or malunion [28].

As Romash used the original fracture to correct the deformity of the malunion, Hansen [29] illustrates a multiplane osteotomy of the calcaneus to address the lateral displacement and shortening of the lateral column. The correction gained by the osteotomy is based upon translation of the calcaneal tuber. Varus or valgus deformity is corrected by medial or lateral translation of the tuber fragment, and calcaneal height is corrected by plantar translation of the tuber. The lateral column lengthening is achieved by the angle with which the anterolateral to posteromedial osteotomy is made. The subtalar joint can be spared with this procedure because the osteotomy is done just posterior to the joint (Fig. 3).

Using their classification system of calcaneal malunions, Stephens and Sanders [23] developed an algorithm for treatment of these malunions. Type I malunions, isolated lateral wall exostosis and pain, were treated with an aggressive lateral wall exostectomy and peroneal tenolysis. Type II malunions, lateral wall impingement with subtalar arthrosis, were treated with a lateral wall exostectomy, peroneal tenolysis, and subtalar arthrodesis using local bone graft from the exostectomy. Type III malunions, lateral wall impingement with subtalar arthrosis and greater than 10 degrees of varus malunion, were treated with lateral wall exostectomy, subtalar arthrodesis, and a calcaneal osteotomy. In their original series, 7 of 7 type I malunions had an excellent [6] or good result [1]. Of the type II malunions, there were 11 excellent, 3 good, and 1 fair result with all patients having the expected difficulty walking on uneven ground due to the subtalar fusion. The type III malunions only had 1 excellent, 1 good, and 2 fair results. There were no malunions or nonunions in this study [23]. Clare and colleagues [30] conducted a study with a longer average follow up of 5.3 years in 45 feet. They achieved union in 93% of the patients undergoing arthrodesis and 42 of 45 (93%) had a neutral to slight valgus hindfoot. All the patients had a plantigrade foot, and 29 patients (64%) had mild residual pain, with 19 having pain in the lateral aspect of the ankle. The American Orthopaedic Foot and Ankle Society ankle and hindfoot scores, Short Form 36 or the Maryland Foot Score did not demonstrate any significant difference between the types of malunions with regard to outcome and function. The authors encountered a rate of 24% delayed wound healing with only one deep infection, and ultimately came to the conclusion that although the protocol did produce acceptable results for the salvage of malunions, acute operative fixation of the fractures may provide more benefit than delayed reconstruction (Fig. 4).

Nonunion of calcaneal fractures

The nonunion rate of primary calcaneal fracture is difficult to determine in the literature due to its low incidence. Nonunions develop when the

biologic environment for healing, such as vascularity and soft tissue coverage, is poor or the method of immobilization or fixation is inadequate. The
calcaneus itself is a well-vascularized bone. Its soft tissue coverage at times
may be tenuous but the osseous structures are well vascularized. With regard to fixation of calcaneus fractures, no matter which method is employed, the fractures are effectively immobilized in short leg casts that
eliminate any motion at either the subtalar or calcaneocuboid joints. Herscovici and colleagues [31] studied operative treatment for 144 calcaneal
fractures in elderly patients (>65 y/o) and only had one nonunion. Zwipp
and colleagues [32] reported a nonunion rate of 1.3% in 123 calcaneal fractures that were operatively managed. Two randomized controlled trials of
operative and nonoperative treatment of calcaneus fractures by Buckley

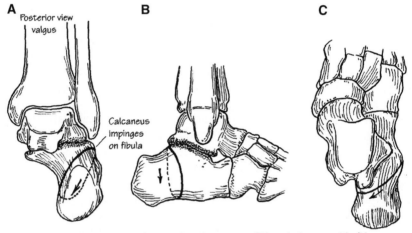

New union stabilized with 6.5 cancellous bone screws; 3.5 cortical screws with glide
holes at right angle to osteotomy; cancellous chips in talo-calcaneal joint

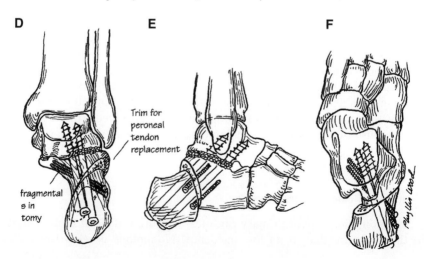

and colleagues [33] (424 patients) and Thordason and Krieger [34] (30 patients) reported no nonunions. Thus, the literature specific to nonunion of calcaneus fractures is nonexistent.

Summary

Though the debate continues between operative interventions versus conservative therapy, there is significant evidence that the deformity that results from calcaneus malunions causes significant disability for the patient. Knowledge of the fracture patterns in the original calcaneal fracture aids in both understanding the deformity of the malunion and the necessary steps for correction of the deformity. Increased heel width, subfibular impingement, tibiotalar impingement, varus/valgus deformity of the hindfoot, peroneal tendon dysfunction, and subtalar arthrosis are all established consequences of calcaneal malunion. Different surgical options have been postulated either trying to address all the deformities or concentrating on certain aspects that are most clinically pressing. The simplest form of treatment is isolated lateral wall decompression, and if applied to a patient who has minimal subtalar arthrosis and no hindfoot deformity, good results are produced. The more complex surgical interventions aim to correct the lateral ankle symptoms, subtalar arthrosis, and hindfoot varus. These surgeries result in a more functional foot but should be considered a salvage procedure because there is still considerable disability as indicated by lower functional scores on the Short Form 36 and American Orthopaedic Foot and

Fig. 3. Calcaneal osteotomy in multiple planes for correction of major posttraumatic deformity. (*A*) Posterior illustration shows sequelae of old calcaneal fracture, including subtalar arthrosis, lateral displacement of the posterior heel, and impingement under the fibula. Curved line depicts the osteotomy. (*B*) Lateral illustration depicts subtalar arthrosis, loss of height at the heel, and shortening of the lateral column. The osteotomy is at the back of the subtalar joint. From this perspective, the cut appears almost vertical. The normal weight-bearing area of the tuber is left undisturbed. When the posterior fragment is mobilized, it will carry with it the attachment of the plantar fascia, the tendo Achillis, and the ground reaction force. (*C*) Dorsoplantar illustration shows the angle of the osteotomy. The cuts are configured to lengthen the lateral column during medial translation. In this example, 10 mm of medial displacement gains approximately 6 or 7 mm of length. (*D*) The tuber has been moved in a medial, plantar, and posterior direction, and subtalar fusion has been performed. The screws are perpendicular to the osteotomy, and two 6.5 mm screws are perpendicular to the subtalar joint. Lag screws are used because the subtalar joint has not been distracted. If distraction is desirable and has been accomplished with a block graft, use of fully threaded screws would be indicated. (*E*) Lateral illustration shows the position of the screws. The plantar and longitudinal displacement of the posterior fragment is apparent. Height is restored. (*F*) Dorsoplantar view shows medial displacement of the tuber fragment and exostectomy of the lateral protrusion. The amount of bone removed by means of the exostectomy can vary, but it must be sufficient to clear the underside of the fibula before the peroneal tendons are replaced. Lateral column length for heel lever arm is restored. (*From* Hansen ST. Functional Reconstruction of the Foot and Ankle. Philadelphia: Lippincot Williams and Wilkins; 2000. p. 383; with permission.)

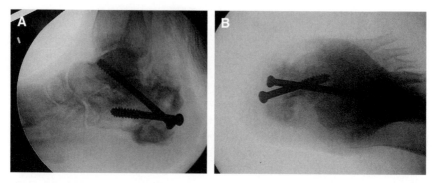

Fig. 4. (*A*) Lateral view of subtalar arthrodesis for Sanders type III calcaneal malunion. Correction of talar declination angle. (*B*) Axial view of subtalar arthrodesis with correction of hindfoot varus and lateral wall exostosis.

Ankle Society hindfoot surveys. Nonunion in calcaneal fractures has limited incidence within the literature for both operative and nonoperative management. Thus, any conclusion as to why there would be such a low incidence can only be made on speculation that the vascularity of the calcaneus and ability to immobilize both the subtalar and calcaneocuboid joints allow the fracture to heal.

References

[1] Lindsay W, Dewar F. Fractures of the os calcis. Am J Surg 1958;95:555–76.
[2] Sanders R. Displaced intra-articular fractures of the calcaneus. J Bone Joint Surg Am 2000; 82:225–50.
[3] Cotton FJ. Fractures of the os calcis. Boston Medical Surgical Journal 1908;18:559–65.
[4] Conn HR. The treatment of fractures of the os calcis. J Bone Joint Surg 1935;17:392–405.
[5] Gallie WE. Subastragalar arthrodesis in fractures of the os calcis. J Bone Joint Surg 1943;25: 731–6.
[6] Hall RL, Shereff MJ. Anatomy of the calcaneus. Clin Orthop 1993;290:27–35.
[7] Harty M. Anatomic consideration in injuries of the calcaneus. Orthop Clin North Am 1973; 4(1):179–83.
[8] Sabry FF, Ebraheim NA, Mehalik JN, et al. Internal architecture of the calcaneus: implications for calcaneus fractures. Foot Ankle Int 2000;21(2):114–8.
[9] Wood Jones F. Buchanan's manual of anatomy, 8th edition. London: Bailliere, Tindall and Cox; 1953. p. 353.
[10] Essex Lopresti P. The mechanism, reduction technique, and results in fractures of the os calcis. Br J Surg 1952;39:395–419.
[11] Bohler L. Diagnosis, pathology and treatment of fractures of the os calcis. J Bone Joint Surg 1931;13:75–89.
[12] Carr, James. Mechanism and pathoanatomy of the intraarticular calcaneal fracture. Clin Orthop 1993;290:36–40.
[13] Mulcahy DM, McCormack DM, Stephens MM. Intra-articular calcaneal fractures: effect of open reduction and internal fixation on the contact characteristics of the subtalar joint. Foot Ankle 1998;19:842–8.
[14] Sangeorzan BJ, Ananthakrishnan D, Tencer AF. Contact characteristics of the subtalar joint after a simulated calcaneus fracture. J Orthop Trauma 1995;9:251–8.

[15] Carr JB, Hamilton JJ, Bear LS. Experimental intra-articular calcaneal fractures: anatomic basis for a new classification. Foot Ankle 1989;10:81–7.

[16] Isbister JF. Clacaneo-fibular abutment following crush fractures of the calcaneus. J Bone Joint Surg [Br] 1974;56b:274–8.

[17] Braly GW, Bishop JO, Tullos HS. Lateral decompression for malunited os calcis fractures. Foot Ankle 1985;6(2):90–2.

[18] Lindsay WRN, Dewar FP. Fractures of the os calcis. Am J Surg 1958;95:555–76.

[19] Carr JB, Hansen ST, Bernischke SK. Subtalar distraction bone block fusion for late complications of os calcis fractures. Foot Ankle 1988;9(2):81–6.

[20] Aronson J, Nunley J, Frankovitch K. Lateral talocalcaneal angle in assessment of subtalar valgus: follow-up of seventy Grice-Green arthrodeses. Foot Ankle 1983;4:56–63.

[21] Broden B. Roentgen examination of the subtaloid joint in fractures of the calcaneus. Acta Radiol 1949;31:85–91.

[22] Crosby LA, Fitzgibbons T. Intraarticular calcaneal fractures results of closed treatment. Clin Orthop 1993;290:47–54.

[23] Stephens HM, Sanders R. Calcaneal malunions: results of a prognostic computed tomography classification system. Foot Ankle Int 1996;17(7):395–401.

[24] Kitaoka HB, Schaap EJ, Chao EY, et al. Displaced intra-articular fractures of the calcaneus treated non-operatively: clinical results and analysis of motion and ground reaction and temporal forces. J Bone Joint Surg Am 1994;76:1531–40.

[25] Burton D, Olney W, Horton G. Late results of subtalar distraction fusion. Foot Ankle Int 1998;19(4):197–202.

[26] Kalamchi A, Evans J. Posterior subtalar fusion. J Bone Joint Surg Br 1977;59:287–9.

[27] Bednarz PA, Beals TC, Manoli A. Subtalar distraction bone block fusion: an assessment of outcome. Foot Ankle Int 1997;18:785–91.

[28] Romash Michael M. Reconstructive osteotomy of the calcaneus with subtalar arthrodesis for malunited calcaneal fractures. Clin Orthop 1993;290:157–67.

[29] Hansen Sigvard T Jr. Functional reconstruction of the foot and ankle. Philadelphia: Lippincott; 2000. p. 380–3.

[30] Clare MP, Lee WE III, Sanders R. Intermediate to long-term results of a treatment protocol for calcaneal fracture malunions. J Bone Joint Surg 2005;87-A:963–73.

[31] Herscovici D Jr, Widmaier J, Scaduto JM, et al. Operative treatment of calcaneal fractures in elderly patients. J Bone Joint Surg 2005;87:1260–4.

[32] Zwipp H, Tscherne H, Thermann H, et al. Osteosynthesis of displaced intraarticular fractures of the calcaneus: results in 123 cases. Clin Orthop 1993;290:76–86.

[33] Buckley R, Tough S, McCormack R, et al. Operative compared with nonoperative treatment of displaced intra-articular calcaneal fractures: a prospective, randomized, controlled multicenter trial. J Bone Joint Surg 2002;84:1733–44.

[34] Thordarson D, Krieger L. Operative vs. nonoperative treatment of intra-articular fractures of the calcaneus: a prospective randomized trial. Foot Ankle Int 1996;17:2–9.

ELSEVIER
SAUNDERS

Foot Ankle Clin N Am
12 (2007) 137–151

Post Talus Neck Fracture Reconstruction

Erik Calvert, MD, FRCSC,
Alastair Younger, MB, ChB, MSc, ChM, FRCSC*,
Murray Penner, BSc (MEng), MD, FRCSC

*Division of Lower Extremity Reconstruction and Oncology, Department of Orthopaedics,
University of British Columbia, 1144 Burrard Street, Vancouver, BC, Canada V6N 2N4*

Talar injuries present a unique set of challenges because of the precarious blood supply and its special function [1]. Restoring anatomy is extremely important but does not necessarily exclude poor outcome because avascular necrosis, malunion, and posttraumatic arthritis are relatively common sequelae. The reconstructive options for avascular necrosis and posttraumatic arthritis are numerous. Anatomic reduction of varus malunions is an effective treatment in the face of normal adjacent joints.

History

The first documentation of a talus injury is from 1608 described by Fabricius of Hilden [2]. Subsequent case reports followed and finally a series of 18 cases was reported in 1919 by H.G. Anderson [3]. The term aviator's astragalus became associated with this injury. The pilots in Anderson's series often had a foot on the rudder and subsequently suffered an extreme hyperdorsiflexion force resulting in a talar neck injury. Coltart's article [4] also described an association with flying accidents. Presently, high-energy injuries involving motor vehicle accidents and falls from height are common mechanisms [5]. Peterson and colleagues [6] found that a combination of axial and dorsiflexion forces was required to produce a talar neck fracture. Daniels and Smith [7] described direct hits, extreme dorsally direct force, and supination with talar neck hitting the medial malleolus as mechanisms of talar neck fractures. Likely the variation in fracture patterns observed

---

* Corresponding author.
E-mail address: asyounger@shaw.ca (A. Younger).

1083-7515/07/$ - see front matter © 2007 Elsevier Inc. All rights reserved.
doi:10.1016/j.fcl.2006.12.006

depends on the degree of eversion and inversion also. This can be deduced from the occasional malleolar fracture associated with talar neck fractures. In their case report, Montane and Zych [8] discuss a Hawkins III talar neck fracture with an associated ipsilateral bimalleolar fracture. Hawkins [9] found 15 of 57 patients had associated fractures of the medial malleolus. Canale and Kelly [10] had similar observations.

Talus fractures compose 1% of all fractures and talar neck fractures make up 50% of these injuries. Our understanding of talar neck injuries has improved; however, dreaded complications persist. Infection, skin necrosis, avascular necrosis, delayed union, nonunion, malunion, and secondary osteoarthritis are implicated problems. These complications result in extremely poor function, chronic pain, stiffness, and revision surgical interventions [11–15]. Hawkins [9] described three different groups of talar neck fractures based on prereduction radiographs. Canale and Kelly [10] added a fourth type, which involved a talonavicular dislocation.

Talar neck fracture complications

Soft tissue

Given the usual high energy of the injury, the fragile soft tissue envelope of the hindfoot is easily compromised. Up to 77% of cases have associated soft tissue complications, such as infection, wound dehiscence, and skin necrosis [16,17]. A soft-tissue injury, from skin tenting to a compound wound, negatively impacts the outcome. Initial management involves irrigation, debridement, and open reduction internal fixation (ORIF) of the fracture with care to avoid further compromising the vascularity of the talus. The injured, avascular talar body can harbor infection easily. If subsequent infection develops, a thorough debridement and irrigation can result in talectomy and subsequent tibiocalcaneal fusion to re-establish some function [18–20]. The other options for fusion are Blair-type and allograft interposition tibiocalcaneal fusion.

Avascular necrosis

Avascular necrosis is a well-known complication of talar neck fractures. The incidence has been found to increase with the energy of the injury [17,21]. The rate of osteonecrosis varies according to study but there seems to be a clear association with the class of Hawkins injury [22]. For type I fractures the reported rate ranges from 0% to 13%; Type II has a range of 20% to 50% and Type III/IV ranges from 8% to 100% [4,9,10,14,16,19,23–25]. Regardless of injury class, the principles of emergent treatment remain careful soft tissue handling, anatomic fixation, and rehabilitation. The timing of definitive fixation has been the center of debate. Lindvall and colleagues [26] and Vallier and colleagues [27] showed that delay in treatment did not impact rates of osteonecrosis or collapse. Lindvall and colleagues [26] further qualified that delay in surgery did not impact American Orthopaedic Foot and Ankle Society (AOFAS) hindfoot score, nonunion rate, osteonecrosis rate, and secondary osteoarthritis.

Union and malunion

Delayed union and nonunion occur rarely after talar neck fractures. Lindvall and colleagues [26] demonstrated an 88% union rate. The time to intervention did not seem to matter in their study. Open fractures healed more slowly than closed fractures, and the better the reduction, the better likelihood of uniting. Vallier and colleagues [27] found a 3.3% nonunion rate defined at 3 months. They had one case of delayed union, which eventually healed at 24 weeks without intervention.

Malunion is unfortunately a relatively common problem and varies somewhat according Hawkins class. Class I has had a reported rate of 0% to 10%, class II 0% to 25%, and class III/IV 18% to 27% ([4,10,16,19,23–25]. Anatomic reduction improves chances of good outcome. Miller [28] and Lindvall and colleagues found that anatomic reduction is important to functional outcome. Because of medial comminution, a varus malunion can result and this needs to be considered when choosing fixation in a talar neck fracture. Screw fixation with various trajectories has been the mainstay for talar neck fractures; however, Fleuriau and colleagues [29] found that their plating technique allowed for a more precise anatomic reduction in the face of comminution. Anatomic reduction is therefore essential to prevent the varus malunion.

Arthritic change

Posttraumatic arthritis can occur in the subtalar joint and ankle joint singly or simultaneously. Subtalar arthritis is more common [30]. The cause of posttraumatic osteoarthritis in this setting is multifactorial. Prolonged immobilization, articular damage, and intra-articular malalignment are factors. The inferior aspect of the talus has been found to be damaged in many cases [5]. Immobilization can result in arthrofibrosis and decreased joint lubrication and nutrition. Radiographic changes are seen in up to 69% of cases [30–32]. Hawkins Type 1 fractures have an observed osteoarthritis rate of 0% to 30%, Hawkins Type II 40% to 90%, and Type III/IV 70% to 100% [4,9,10,14,16,19,23–25]. Fig. 1 demonstrates a case of posttraumatic arthritis treated with subtalar arthrodesis.

Diagnosis

History and physical

When seeing a patient who has had a talar neck fracture it is helpful to gain as much information as possible. A full history of the accident,

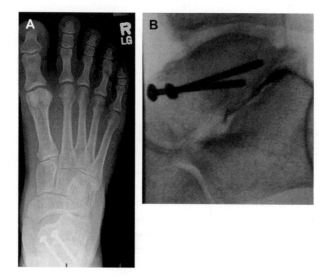

Fig. 1. This patient presents with ongoing pain after a talar neck fracture when he was 12 years old. An open reduction was performed. He did well until recently. Changes were seen in the ankle and subtalar joint. To confirm that the pain was arising from the ankle joint a local anesthetic block was performed. An arthroscopic subtalar fusion was performed with successful outcome. (*A*) Anteroposterior (AP) view of the foot. (*B*) Arthrogram/injection subtalar joint.

mechanism of injury, associated injuries, and treatment to date are needed. Any early or late complications are noted. Previous operative reports, serial radiographs, and relevant consult notes are reviewed. Relevant history includes pain, development of callosities, limb shortening, functional limitations, and change in the shape of the foot.

On physical examination pertinent findings are change in the leg length, ankle range limitation, varus deformity, forefoot adduction, and decreased hindfoot eversion [33]. Fig. 2 demonstrates the typical features of a varus malunion of the talar neck. Daniels and colleagues [33] also demonstrated a lax deltoid ligament resulting from a varus malunion. Furthermore, neurovascular status of the foot and ankle and the status of the overlying integument and previous incisions should be noted.

Investigations

Once the patient is reviewed, further investigations may be required. Standing plain radiographs are inspected. The Hawkins sign for avascular necrosis (AVN) can be a simple indication of osteonecrosis. Henderson [34] described a case of a Hawkins III fracture that was treated with emergent reduction and fixation. Serial MRIs were done that actually did not demonstrate AVN. The patient did not have the Hawkins [9] sign, however, and underwent a core biopsy of his talus, which confirmed AVN. CT scan is

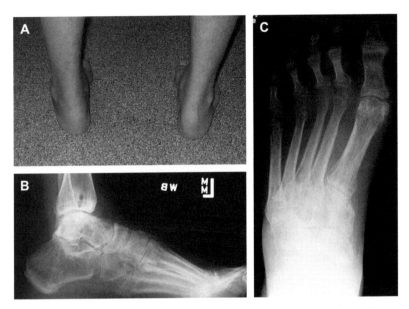

Fig. 2. (*A*) Varus hindfoot alignment. (*B*) Lateral foot and ankle. (*C*) AP foot. Hindfoot varus post talar neck malunion. The patient has a varus left ankle after a Hawkins II talar neck fracture. The fracture has malunited into a dorsiflexed and internally rotated position, which locks the midfoot and can prevent midfoot motion, causing stiffness and pain. This patient would require a subtalar fusion and calcaneocuboid fusion with lateral column shortening to correct the foot position. No reconstruction has been performed to date.

an excellent modality for following union of a fracture compared with plain radiographs. For the most part, however, MRI is good for delineating the extent of AVN in a given talar body. Finally, for those patients in whom infection is suspected, an erythrocyte sedimentation rate and a C-reactive protein should be ordered.

Management of avascular necrosis

Nonoperative

The management of avascular necrosis can be thought of as preventative, emergent, and reconstructive. Many authors have advocated early reduction and fixation of talar neck fractures to prevent avascular necrosis [35–37]. Two recent studies have evidence to suggest otherwise. Lindvall and colleagues [26] and Vallier and colleagues [27] found that delayed reduction and fixation did not adversely affect rates of avascular necrosis. It has been widespread practice to limit weight bearing once AVN is established [38]. Hawkins discussed 9 of 13 patients who had AVN who went on to collapse. He stated that prolonged non–weight bearing to bridge the time of bone substitution is poorly tolerated. The series by Canale and Kelly [10] describes 23 cases of AVN treated nonoperatively. They found that the patients who were non–weight bearing for an average of 8 months faired much better than those who lasted less than 3 months on the crutches. Another study found that extensive non–weight bearing did not prevent talar collapse [39] Often, allowing the patient to weight bear is the best option because it is difficult to be non–weight bearing for a prolonged period of time (Fig. 3). The degree of involvement should be evaluated because not all cases of AVN are alike. When there is partial osteonecrosis, the remainder of the talus can offer support and weight bearing with a brace could be allowed [35]. Once it has been established that prolonged weight bearing has not prevented collapse, reconstructive options come into play.

Reconstruction after avascular necrosis and collapse

Operative options for postcollapse osteonecrosis include talectomy, Blair-type fusion, tibiocalcaneal fusion, pantalar fusion, total ankle arthroplasty, and below knee amputation. Core decompression has been advocated by Mont and colleagues [40] for precollapse talar AVN. Their patients were not posttraumatic and they had 14 of 17 ankles of patients who had been on chronic corticosteroids. It would not be prudent to extrapolate this data to the posttraumatic population. One initial thought was that subtalar arthrodesis may help in promoting revascularization [41]. A few series have described their follow-up of this approach; they did not demonstrate any advantage to early subtalar fusion [10,19]. Talectomy has been performed with poor results [4,9,41–43]. Combining talectomy with tibiocalcaneal fusion has

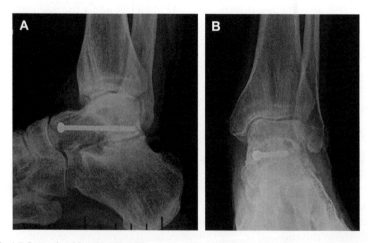

Fig. 3. (A) Lateral ankle. (B) AP ankle. A 34-year-old patient who suffered a Hawkins type III talar neck fracture. An open reduction was performed. He was seen 6 months after for an opinion with regard to activity level to prevent collapse of the talar body. He was mobilized and these radiographs were taken 2.5 years after the injury. He has full function and works as a hot house manager on his feet all day.

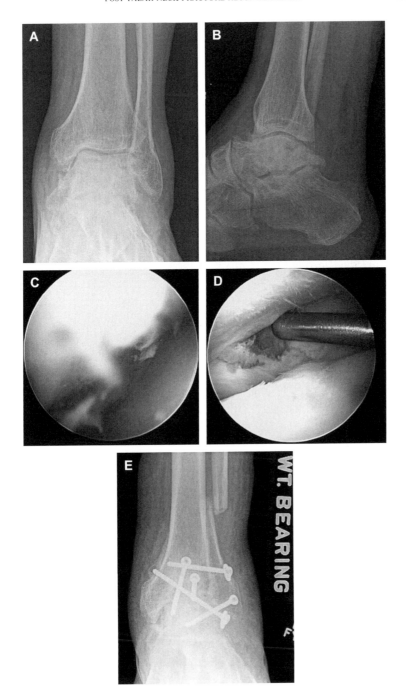

been found to be advantageous [44]. The ability to achieve fusion with a compromised talus is difficult. The tibiocalcaneal fusion allows fusion of two healthy bone surfaces depending on the technique. It has been found by some that tibiocalcaneal fusion has better results than ankle fusion or talectomy [10,19]. Maintenance of limb length and foot shape aid in fitting shoe wear. Reckling [45] found that 15 of 16 patients who had undergone tibiocalcaneal fusion had good results with an average limb shortening of 1.25 in. In a tibiocalcaneal fusion the limb is shorter and the ankle wider, thereby making it problematic to wear shoes. Kitaoka and Patzer (1998) [46] found reliable results after arthrodesis for talar AVN. If retaining foot shape and limb length are a priority then a Blair-type fusion with or without bone graft is done. The Blair-type arthrodesis has had several modifications. Blair [47] described a sliding tibial graft. Thereafter, fixation modifications and structural bone graft have been used [48–50]. The method of fixation varies according to surgeon preference. The Blair-type fusion can lead to abnormal load through the remnant of the subtalar joint. The anterior and middle facets of the subtalar joint are likely to undergo degeneration if they bear the entire load [51]. Kitaoka and colleagues [46] advocate for maintenance of any viable talar body, but if insufficient, then they recommend tibiocalcaneal arthrodesis. They maintain the talar body when possible to maintain limb length and foot shape. Their fusion rate was similar to patients who had uncompromised tali. Nonunion is a common complication post Blair-type reconstruction. Fig. 4 is an example of such a problem. Talar body prostheses have been studied in 16 patients [52]. They reported 10 good results and difficulties in fitting the correct shape of the prosthesis. We have one patient for whom a talar body prosthesis for a total ankle was produced (Fig. 5). He has had an excellent result and has returned to work. This alternative requires further study. Total ankle replacement is an emerging solution for this difficult problem. In patients who have adequate talar body remaining after debridement a total ankle replacement can be used to provide the patient with maintenance of limb length, a chance at improved function, and relief of pain. Fig. 6 demonstrates such an approach in a patient.

◄──

Fig. 4. This patient had a talar neck fracture after a work-related fall. He started to get AVN of the talar body. Ankle and subtalar arthroscopies were performed confirming well-preserved tibial and calcaneal cartilage in the ankle and subtalar joints, respectively. A custom talar body replacement was sought but could not be manufactured in an appropriate time period. The ankle was therefore fused with a modified Blair technique. The patient has developed a symptomatic nonunion and wishes to continue without further surgical treatment. (*A*) AP ankle. (*B*) Lateral ankle. (*C*) Subtalar arthroscopy. (*D*) Ankle arthroscopy. (*E*) Nonunion ankle fusion. Subtalar scope: The talus is superior with degenerative change whereas the calcaneal surface inferiorly is well preserved. Similar changes are seen in the ankle with fissuring of the talar cartilage inferiorly and well-preserved tibial cartilage. Because of the inability to find an appropriate manufacturer of a talar body replacement preserving the talar head we elected to perform a modified Blair fusion. He has gone on to nonunion of this, a recognized complication of this procedure.

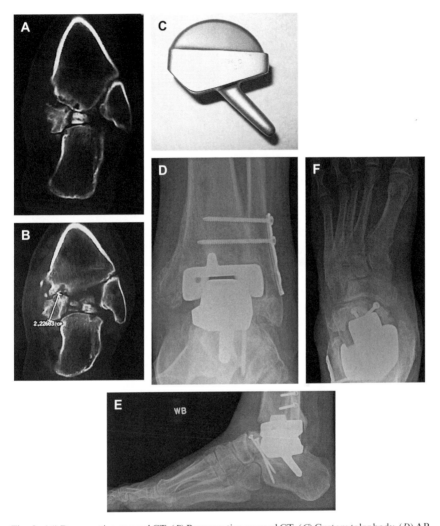

Fig. 5. (*A*) Preoperative coronal CT. (*B*) Preoperative coronal CT. (*C*) Custom talar body. (*D*) AP ankle total ankle replacement. (*E*) Lateral total ankle replacement. (*F*) AP of the foot, total ankle replacement. This 58-year-old mill worker fell in a remote town suffering a Hawkins III talar neck fracture. His surgical management was delayed as a result. His talar body went on to collapse and fragment and his ankle joint became arthritic. After discussion he consented to a custom total ankle with a talar body replacement. He is now 3 years postsurgery and has returned to full-time work.

Reconstruction of malunion without avascular necrosis

Corrective arthrodeses for talar neck malunion and nonunion include subtalar, ankle, talonavicular, and triple arthrodeses. These procedures are effective for deformity correction and pain relief; however, they do eventually result in adjacent joint degeneration [53,54]. Triple arthrodesis has not been shown to be effective for varus neck deformity [10].

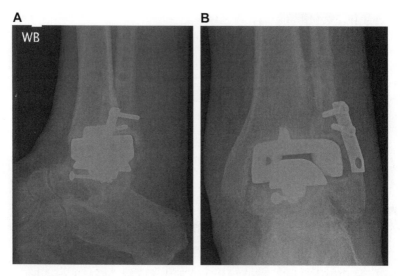

Fig. 6. Patient who has posttraumatic change after a talar neck fracture from a fall from height. He presented 8 years later with increasing ankle joint pain. CT and MRI showed that the body had collapsed and revascularized. A total ankle replacement was therefore performed after the bone was found to be solid and bleeding intraoperatively. A subtalar fusion was also performed. The total ankle replacement was performed 5 years ago and complicated by a fibular fracture 2 years ago requiring ORIF. He has otherwise enjoyed a good outcome from the total ankle arthroplasty. (*A*) Lateral total ankle arthroplasty. (*B*) AP total ankle arthroplasty.

When a patient presents with a malunion of a talar neck fracture, one commonly observes a dorsal displacement or varus deformity. Dorsal displacement can interfere with ankle dorsiflexion. In cases with dorsal displacement, the dorsal beak can be resected to eradicate the impingement in dorsiflexion [10]. A varus malunion causes the talar neck to be short and to be deviated medially and dorsally. This deformity leads to varus through the talonavicular, calcaneocuboid, and subtalar joints [51]. Varus deformity can result in an adducted forefoot, varus hindfoot, and decreased eversion [33]. Consideration of the peritalar articulations should be undertaken. In the absence of adjacent arthroses, anatomic reconstruction of the talar neck malunion can be considered. This reconstruction would offer a chance at normal function, whereas corrective arthrodesis would not. Rammelt and colleagues [55] found excellent results in their series of 10 patients followed for a mean of 4 years; 9 out of 10 cases were satisfied. The 1 that was not required an ankle fusion 8 years postosteotomy. Their mean AOFAS Ankle Hindfoot Score improved from 38 to 86. A case report by Monroe and Manoli [56] described a patient who had a varus deformity post nonoperative treatment of a Hawkins II talar neck fracture. They proceeded with a talar neck osteotomy and interpositional iliac crest bone graft and fixation with a 3.5 mm cortical screw. At 56 months the patient had returned to his preinjury heavy labor job and his AOFAS score increased from 11 to 85. In both of the above reports all osteotomies united and there were no cases of AVN progression noted. Two papers described nonunion surgery without malalignment, which resulted in solid union (Migues and colleagues 1996 [57], and Acencio and colleagues 2000 [58]). In light of these papers the anatomic reconstruction of talar neck malunions is a plausible alternative to corrective arthrodesis. We have treated a patient with a nonunion of his talar neck injury with revision ORIF. He has achieved a good result (Fig. 7).

For correction of a varus malunion or nonunion, the patient is placed supine, a tourniquet is applied, and preoperative antibiotics are administered.

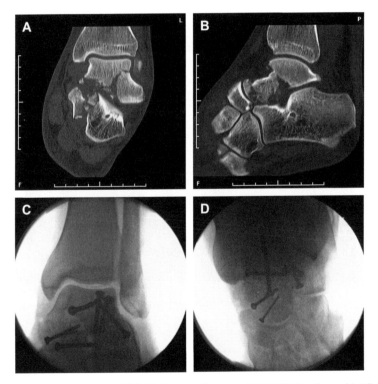

Fig. 7. (*A*) Preoperative coronal CT. (*B*) Preoperative sagittal CT (ORIF radiograph). (*C*) Postoperative ORIF AP ankle. (*D*) Postoperative ORIF AP foot. (*E*) Nonunion talar neck, AP ankle. (*F*) Nonunion talar neck, lateral foot and ankle. (*G*) Postrevision ORIF, lateral foot and ankle. (*H*) Postrevision ORIF, AP foot. (*I*) Postrevision ORIF, oblique foot. This 20-year-old male was in a work-related motorcycle accident. He had talar head and neck fractures and a comminuted sustentaculum injury. He was referred from a distant hospital and treated with ORIF a few days postinjury. Persistent pain 1 year postoperatively resulted in ankle arthroscopy, debridement, and removal of some hardware. Subsequent diagnosis of nonunion was made. Open debridement, interpositional autologous bone graft, and revision fixation were undertaken. He has had an excellent result clinically and radiographically. Preoperative coronal CT and sagittal CT.

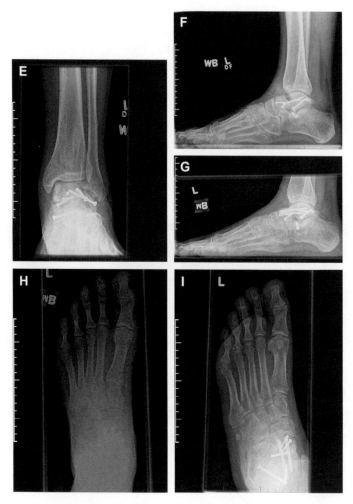

Fig. 7 (*continued*)

The limb and the ipsilateral crest are prepped and draped. The corrective site can be approached through an anteromedial approach between tibialis anterior and tibialis posterior. The fracture malunion or nonunion site is exposed and the fracture line is recreated carefully. A small laminar spreader is interposed to provisionally reduce the deformity. Once the reduction is achieved, the interpositional graft is fashioned from the iliac crest. This graft is shaped and interposed. Radiographs with provisional fixation and graft are taken. Adjacent symptomatic joints are addressed. Definitive fixation is then introduced. Final radiographs are taken. Meticulous soft tissue handling is of the utmost importance during closure. A postoperative non–weight-bearing splint is fabricated for 10 days. A wound check is performed and if satisfactory then range of motion is started. Weight bearing begins when union is evident.

Summary

Talar neck fractures are interesting fractures that require careful ORIF if the patient factors allow. The long-term sequelae of these fractures can be severe regardless of the quality of the reconstruction. Posttraumatic arthritis and avascular necrosis are devastating complications that are unfortunately common. Malunion and nonunion of talar neck fractures need to be evaluated carefully with attention to adjacent joints. A full workup is needed to fully evaluate the patient and fracture factors. If the patient has failed nonoperative treatment then reconstruction or salvage is considered. Reconstruction of ununited and malunited talar neck fractures can be successful if the patient is well selected. Corrective fusion is a viable alternative for those patients who have posttraumatic arthritis. Combined ankle replacement and subtalar fusion remains another motion-conserving procedure.

References

[1] Baumhauer JF, Alvarez RG. Controversies in treating talus fractures. Orthop Clin North Am 1995;26(2):335–51.

[2] Bonnin JG. Dislocations and fracture dislocations of te talus. Br J Surg 1940;28:88–100.

[3] Anderson HG. The medical and surgical aspects of aviation. London: Oxford University Press; 1919.

[4] Coltart WD. Aviator's astragalus. J Bone Joint Surg Br 1952;34:545–66.

[5] Sanders DW. Fractures of the talus; Fractures in adults. ed. RW Bucholz, Heckman JD, Court-Brown CM. vol. 6. Philadelphia: Lippincott Williams and Wilkins 2006. p. 2249–92.

[6] Peterson L, Romanus B, Dahlberg E. Fracture of the collum tali—an experimental study. J Biomech 1976;9(4):277–9.

[7] Daniels TR, Smith JW. Foot fellow's review. Foot Ankle Int 1993;14:225–34.

[8] Montane I, Zych GA. An unusual fracture of the talus associated with a bimalleolar ankle fracture. A case report and review of the literature. Clin Orthop Relat Res 1986;July(208): 278–81.

[9] Hawkins LG. Fractures of the neck of the talus. J Bone Joint Surg Am 1970;52(5):991–1002.

[10] Canale ST, Kelly FB Jr. Fractures of the neck of the talus. Long-term evaluation of seventy-one cases. J Bone Joint Surg Am 1978;60(2):143–56.

[11] Mindell ER, Cisek EE, Kartalian G, et al. Late results of injuries to the talus. Analysis of forty cases. J Bone Joint Surg Am 1963;45:221–45.

[12] Archdeacon M, Wilber R. Fractures of the talar neck. Orthop Clin North Am 2002;33(1): 247–62.

[13] Higgins TF, Baumgaertner MR. Diagnosis and treatment of fractures of the talus: a comprehensive review of the literature. Foot Ankle Int 1999;20(9):595–605.

[14] Santavirta S, Seitsalo S, Kiviluoto O, et al. Fractures of the talus. J Trauma 1984;24(11): 986–9.

[15] Szyszkowitz R, Reschauer R, Seggl W. Eighty-five talus fractures treated by ORIF with five to eight years of follow-up study of 69 patients. Clin Orthop Relat Res 1985;October(199): 97–107.

[16] Kenwright J, Taylor RG. Major injuries of the talus. J Bone Joint Surg Br 1970;52(1):36–48.

[17] Gilquist J, Oretop N, Stenstrom A, et al. Late results after vertical fracture of the talus. Injury 1974;6(2):173–9.

[18] Omer GEJ, Pomeranz GM. Inital management of severe open injuries and traumatic amputations of the foot. Arch Surg 1972;105:696–8.

[19] Pennal GF. Fractures of the talus. Clin Orthop Relat Res 1963;30:53–63.

[20] Pantazopoulos T, Galanos P, Vayanos E, et al. Fractures of the neck of the talus. Acta Orthop Scand 1974;45(2):296–306.

[21] Behrens F, Long term results of displaced talar neck fractures. Major fractures of the pilon, the talus and the calcaneus: current concepts of treatment. Tscherne HS, Schatzker J, editors. Berlin: Springer-Verlag; 1993. p. 113–21.

[22] Metzger MJ, Levin JS, Clancy JT. Talar neck fractures and rates of avascular necrosis. J Foot Ankle Surg 1999;38(2):154–62.

[23] Boyd HB, Knight RA. Fractures of the astragalus. South Med J 1942;35:160–7.

[24] Grob D, Simpson LA, Weber BG, et al. Operative treatment of displaced talus fractures. Clin Orthop Relat Res 1985;October(199):88–96.

[25] Marsh JL, Saltzman CL, Iverson M, et al. Major open injuries of the talus. J Orthop Trauma 1995;9(5):371–6.

[26] Lindvall E, Haidukewych G, DiPasquale T, et al. Open reduction and stable fixation of isolated, displaced talar neck and body fractures. J Bone Joint Surg Am 2004;86-A(10): 2229–34.

[27] Vallier HA, Nork SE, Barei DP, et al. Talar neck fractures: results and outcomes. J Bone Joint Surg Am 2004;86-A(8):1616–24.

[28] Miller WE. Operative intervention for fracture of the talus., Foot and ankle. ed. JE Bateman, Trott AW. New York:Decker; 1980. p. 52–63.

[29] Fleuriau Chateau PB, Brokaw DS, Jelen BA, et al. Plate fixation of talar neck fractures: preliminary review of a new technique in twenty-three patients. J Orthop Trauma 2002;16(4): 213–9.

[30] Sanders DW, Busam M, Hattwick E, et al. Functional outcomes following displaced talar neck fractures. J Orthop Trauma 2004;18(5):265–70.

[31] Elgafy H, Ebraheim NA, Tile M, et al. Fractures of the talus: experience of two level 1 trauma centers. Foot Ankle Int 2000;21(12):1023–9.

[32] Schulze W, Richter J, Russe O, et al. Surgical treatment of talus fractures: a retrospective study of 80 cases followed for 1–15 years. Acta Orthop Scand 2002;73(3):344–51.

[33] Daniels TR, Smith JW, Ross TI. Varus malalignment of the talar neck. Its effect on the position of the foot and on subtalar motion. J Bone Joint Surg Am 1996;78(10):1559–67.

[34] Henderson RC. Posttraumatic necrosis of the talus: the Hawkins sign versus magnetic resonance imaging. J Orthop Trauma 1991;5(1):96–9.

[35] Comfort TH, Behrens F, Gaither DW, et al. Long-term results of displaced talar neck fractures. Clin Orthop Relat Res 1985;October(199):81–7.

[36] Frawley PA, Hart JA, Young DA. Treatment outcome of major fractures of the talus. Foot Ankle Int 1995;16(6):339–45.

[37] Grob D, Weber BG, Simpson LA. [Trauma-induced necrosis of the corpus tali]. Unfallchirurg 1985;88(4):175–81.

[38] Adelaar RS, Madrian JR. Avascular necrosis of the talus. Orthop Clin North Am 2004; 35(3):383–95.

[39] Penny JN, Davis LA. Fractures and fracture-dislocations of the neck of the talus. J Trauma 1980;20(12):1029–37.

[40] Mont MA, Schon LC, Hungerford MW, et al. Avascular necrosis of the talus treated by core decompression. J Bone Joint Surg Am 1996;78:827–30.

[41] McKeever FM. Treatment of complications of fractures and dislocations of the talus. Clin Orthop Relat Res 1963;30:45–52.

[42] Dunn AR, Jacobs B, Campbell RD Jr. Fractures of the talus. J Trauma 1966;6(4): 443–68.

[43] Pennal GF, Yadav MP. Operative treatment of comminuted fractures of the Os calcis. Orthop Clin North Am 1973;4(1):197–211.

[44] Detenbeck LC, Kelly PJ. Total dislocation of the talus. J Bone Joint Surg Am 1969;51(2): 283–8.

[45] Reckling FW. Early tibiocalcaneal fusion in the treatment of severe injuries of the talus. J Trauma 1972;12(5):390–6.

[46] Kitaoka HB, Patzer GL. Arthrodesis for the treatment of arthrosis of the ankle and osteonecrosis of the talus. J Bone Joint Surg Am 1998;80(3):370–9.

[47] Blair HC. Comminuted fractures and fracture dislocations of the body of the astragalus. Operative treatment. Am J Surg 1943;59:37–43.

[48] Lionberger DR, Bishop JO, Tullos HS. The modified Blair fusion. Foot Ankle 1982;3(1): 60–2.

[49] Morris HD. Aseptic necrosis of the talus following injury. Orthop Clin North Am 1974;5(1): 177–89.

[50] Morris HD, Hand WL, Dunn AW. The modified Blair fusion for fractures of the talus. J Bone Joint Surg Am 1971;53(7):1289–97.

[51] Sangeorzan BJ, Wagner UA, Harrington RM, et al. Contact characteristics of the subtalar joint: the effect of talar neck misalignment. J Orthop Res 1992;10:544–51.

[52] Harnroongroj T, Vanadurongwan V. The talar body prosthesis. J Bone Joint Surg Am 1997; 79(9):1313–22.

[53] Fuchs S, Sandman C, Skwara A, et al. Quality of life 20 years after arthrodesis of the ankle. A study of adjacents joints. J Bone Joint Surg Br 2003;85:994–8.

[54] Coester LM, Saltzman CL, Leopold J, et al. Long term results following ankle arthrodesis for post-traumatic arthritis. J Bone Joint Surg Am 2001;83:219–28.

[55] Rammelt S, Winkler J, Heineck J, et al. Anatomical reconstruction of malunited talus fractures: a prospective study of 10 patients followed for 4 years. Acta Orthop 2005;76(4): 588–96.

[56] Monroe MT, Manoli A. Osteotomy for malunion of a talar neck fracture: a case report. Foot Ankle Int 1999;20(3):192–5.

[57] Migues A, Solari G, Carrasco NM, et al. Repair of talar neck nonunion with indirect corticocancellous graft technique: a case report and review of the literature. Foot Ankle Int 1996; 17(11):690–4.

[58] Asencio G, Rebai M, Bertin R, et al. [Pseudarthrosis and non-union of disjunctive talar fractures]. Rev Chir Orthop Reparatrice Appar Mot 2000;86(2):173–80.

ELSEVIER
SAUNDERS

Foot Ankle Clin N Am
12 (2007) 153–176

FOOT AND
ANKLE CLINICS

Reconstruction of the Varus Ankle from Soft-Tissue Procedures with Osteotomy Through Arthrodesis

Susan Mosier LaClair, MD[a,b]

[a]Department of Orthopaedic Surgery, Michigan State University,
East Lansing, MI 48824, USA
[b]Family Orthopedic Associates, 4466 West Bristol Road, Flint, MI 48507, USA

There are many etiologies of the cavovarus foot and ankle [1]. The subtle cavus foot is thought to be idiopathic and hereditary, with no clear genetic determinants, and may vary in severity from generation to generation. The obvious neurological causes range from Charcot-Marie-Tooth disease to other central and peripheral nerve disorders, including polio, cerebrovascular accident, spinal cord neoplasm, and herniated nucleus pulposus. Post-traumatic cavovarus foot and ankle deformity may arise from complications related to calcaneus or talus fractures as well as tranverse tarsal joint or midfoot fracture dislocations. Compartment syndromes and the resulting scarred muscle may also lead to this deformity [2]. A malunion of a pilon or distal tibiofibular ankle fracture can result in a varus ankle joint or varus overloaded joint [3]. Other known etiologies of the cavovarus foot and ankle include talipes equinovarus, and less commonly, rheumatoid arthritis or talocalcaneal and calcaneonavicular tarsal coalitions [4].

Biomechanics of the cavovarus foot

There are many common characteristics of a cavovarus foot that over time may lead to a varus ankle. Most patients have a combination of one or more of the following traits: plantarflexion of the first or multiple metatarsals, a varus heel, forefoot adduction, supination or pronation, a tight gastroc-Achilles complex, or plantar aponeurosis, with or without clawing of the greater and lesser toes [5,6]. Over time these anatomic variations

E-mail address: marksuelaclair@msn.com

1083-7515/07/$ - see front matter © 2007 Elsevier Inc. All rights reserved.
doi:10.1016/j.fcl.2006.12.008

can lead to symptoms of metatarsalgia, lateral column overload with or without lateral ankle instability, midfoot arthritis, hindfoot arthritis, and eventually a varus malaligned ankle with osteoarthritis [7].

Plantarflexed metatarsals cause increased pressure of the metatarsal phalyngeal joints and often metatarsalgia. Clawing of the metatarsal phalyngeal joints may exacerbate this problem by holding the metatarsal heads in a plantarflexed position. The plantarflexed metatarsals may lead to supination of the forefoot and lateral column overload, resulting in stress fractures of the lateral metatarsals and lateral ankle or subtalar joint instability [5]. Increased plantarflexion of the first metatarsal may result in forefoot valgus or pronation, which places an inversion torque against the calcaneus to create a plantigrade forefoot [7]. This can also lead to lateral ankle or subtalar joint instability, especially if peroneal muscle weakness is present. The subtle cavus foot is thought to result as a primary deformity of the plantarflexed first ray [6]. A plantarflexed first metatarsal will strike the ground first during foot flat and heel rise portions of the gait cycle, resulting in the inability of the subtalar and midfoot joints to evert after heel strike, tipping the foot and ankle into varus. An overactive peroneus longus may act to increase plantarflexion of the first ray, exacerbating this problem. Initially, this deformity is flexible, but with time it can become stiff and then rigid, leading to a fixed hindfoot or heel varus.

In longstanding cavovarus foot and ankle deformity, the progressive rigidity of the deformity can result in contracture of the plantar aponeurosis and equines contracture of the gastroc-Achilles complex, further reinforcing the deformities [8]. Clinically, most patients are observed to have a tight gastrocnemius muscle. This is evaluated using the Silverskiöld test [9]. The ankle is dorsiflexed during knee flexion and extension. If the patient has no ankle dorsiflexion passively above neutral with the knee extended and can obtain ankle dorsiflexion of 5° with the knee flexed, this demonstrates gastrocnemius tightness. This tightness and the resulting ankle plantarflexion can lead to a mechanical advantage for the peroneus longus tendon on the first ray versus its antagonist, the anterior tibial tendon. This muscle imbalance has been proposed to be one of the reasons for worsening of a cavovarus foot and ankle deformity over time [8].

Evaluation of cavovarus deformity

In the treatment of the cavovarus foot and ankle it is important to evaluate if the deformity is flexible or rigid. This is ascertained using a Coleman block test [10]. This is performed by first observing the patient standing from behind and noting the amount of heel varus. The patient's standing foot is then placed on a one inch block of wood, with the great toe and the first metatarsal head off the medial side of the block, along with the medial one quarter of the heel. If there is improvement of the heel varus to a normal slight valgus position, this reveals that the subtalar joint is flexible, and that the plantarflexed first ray is a contributing factor behind the heel varus. Therefore, the Coleman block test is a determination of forefoot-driven hindfoot varus with a flexible deformity.

It is also important to determine the apex of the deformity that you are treating in order to choose the appropriate surgical treatment. Cavus deformity can be driven from the hindfoot, midfoot, or forefoot, or a combination of all three. In hindfoot cavus, there is a dorsiflexed calcaneus in which the pitch of the calcaneus will be greater then 30° [11]. In midfoot cavus, the apex of the deformity falls between the anterior process calcaneus and the medial cuneiform. In forefoot cavus, the apex of the deformity is at the tarsometatarsal joints, with the primary cause being plantarflexion of the first metatarsal.

To assist in the presurgical evaluation of the cavovarus foot, standing radiographs of the foot and ankle should be obtained. Because it is important to compare with what is normal for the patient, bilateral weight-bearing radiographs should be done. These usually consist of anteroposterior (AP) or mortise ankle views, a lateral view of the foot and ankle, combined with an AP foot view. If both feet or ankles can be placed on one cassette for side-to-side comparison, this is very helpful. The standing AP or mortise ankle views allow assessment of joint alignment, neutral versus varus, and the presence of any pre-existing osteoarthritis. The talus appears externally rotated in the mortise with a posterior fibular position [11]. If the patient has a greater cavovarus deformity on one side compared with the other, a difference in the standing ankle height can be observed and quantified [12].

Weight-bearing AP radiographs of the foot can demonstrate a stacking or overlapping of the metatarsals secondary to hindfoot varus with a decreased talocalaneal angle. Some patients will display metatarsus adductus as well [11]. Often midfoot osteoarthritis is seen from a longstanding cavus foot. Stress fractures or cortical thickening of the metatarsal neck or shafts from chronic forefoot overload may be noted [7]. Jones fractures of the fifth metatarsal can also be present from lateral column overload. Subluxation or dislocation of the metatarsal phalyngeal joints from claw toes or intrinsic weakness can be identified in the forefoot, as well as congenitally long lesser metatarsals, which can contribute to metatarsalgia [11].

The lateral foot and ankle view can be used to assess first ray plantarflexion by looking for a disruption of Meary's line from the talus to the tarsal bones to the first metatarsal [11]. This view can also be used to quantify the high or cavus arch, by measuring the increased distance between the medial cuneiform and the fifth metatarsal bases, or a dorsiflexed calcaneus as previously described [7,11,12]. At the ankle, a posterior fibula with respect to the distal tibia is observed, and osteoarthritis of the ankle or hindfoot joints may be noted [11,13].

Other studies that may be required are bilateral AP stress inversion stress test and lateral anteroposterior stress test radiographs to identify lateral ankle instability. Hindfoot alignment views have been described by

Saltzman and El-Koury [14] to evaluate hindfoot varus. These have also been used by Fortin and colleagues [15] as a quantitative Coleman block test. The hindfoot alignment view is taken with and without a half inch block beneath the lateral hindfoot and forefoot with weight-bearing AP ankle radiographs. These views assess the flexibility of the hindfoot or the contribution of forefoot valgus and first ray plantarflexion to the hindfoot varus. If the ankle varus reduces or improves with the Coleman block radiographically, this indicates a flexible deformity.

An MRI of the ankle may be necessary in this same patient population to rule out a coexisting osteochondritis dissecans lesion of the talus or a peroneal tendon tear, and to confirm instability or ligamentous disruption. In rare patients, a CT scan may be warranted to identify or rule out a tarsal coalition. Scranton and colleagues [13] described a malleolar index to objectively measure a posteriorly positioned fibula using axial CT scan images.

Nonoperative treatment

Once the patient's cavovarus foot and ankle has been properly evaluated and the specific problems identified, nonoperative intervention can be initiated. Though this does not cure the problem of the cavovarus foot, it can offer significant symptomatic relief in many patients, especially those who have a flexible deformity. This treatment usually consists of an aggressive gastroc-Achilles stretching program with the use of an orthotic or brace [7]. This should be undertaken for at least 3 to 6 months to see its maximal efficacy. For those patients who have ankle instability, a physical therapy program for strengthening, stretching, and proprioceptive retraining with the use of a sports-type brace for uneven ground or sports activities is also required in addition to orthotic treatment. If the nonoperative management fails to provide adequate pain relief, then operative treatment is undertaken.

Traditionally the cavovarus foot and ankle has been treated with a full-length custom orthotic with a medial arch support high enough for the patient's cavus deformity, with a recess under the first metatarsal head and a graduated lateral wedge, with or without a metatarsal pad. Though this will work for many patients to relieve their symptoms of lateral column or forefoot overload, some patients will require a different type of cavus orthotic. A new prefabricated Cavusfoot Orthotic (Archrival, DJO Incorporated, Vista, CA) has been made available that features an elevated heel, a recess under the first metatarsal head, and a lateral forefoot wedge starting just lateral to the first metatarsal recess, combined with a reduced medial arch height [7]. This is proposed to accommodate a tight gastrocnemius muscle, and allow for the plantarflexed first ray and forefoot pronation, while encouraging hindfoot varus to a more neutral position.

In patients who have a rigid cavovarus deformity, orthotic treatment may still be beneficial for offloading painful areas depending on their complaints;

however, a large majority of these patients have painful osteoarthritic ankle, hindfoot, or midfoot joints, and will require custom bracing with a soft orthotic interface. The goal for these patients is a stable, braceable plantigrade foot and ankle with decreased pain and without skin breakdown. In most of these patients a custom ankle foot orthosis (AFO) is obtained, with an accommodative cavus-type orthotic in it.

The cavovarus foot with lateral ankle instability and its relationship to osteoarthritis

Once a fixed cavovarus foot deformity occurs, it can alter biomechanical contact stresses through the ankle joint and its adjacent hindfoot and midfoot joints [15,16]. The ankle is relatively resistant to primary osteoarthritis, but its thin articular cartilage and decreased contact area can predispose to high peak contact stresses [17]. Long-term ankle incongruency or instability presumably increases ankle contact stress that exceeds the capacity of the ankle joint to repair or adapt itself, leading to osteoarthritis. Ramsey and Hamilton [18] found that shifting the talus 1 mm decreased the contact area of the ankle by 42% and increased the contact stress twofold. When forces are altered across the joint, such as with varus tilt of the talus, distal tibia, or calcaneus, with or without chronic ankle instability, this can lead to degenerative arthritis [7,13,15,19–23].

Cavovarus foot and ankle deformity has been reported to be more frequent in patients who have lateral ankle instability [7,13,15,19–22]. Several authors have confirmed the presence of limb, heel, or ankle joint varus deformity in association with chronic ankle instability. Sugimoto and colleagues [20] compared a group of 85 patients who had chronic ankle instability to acute injuries and normal volunteers. The chronically unstable patients were found to have a significantly greater incidence of varus inclination of the tibial plafond. The study authors proposed that a varus hindfoot or a varus tibial plafond is a possible predisposing factor toward chronic ankle instability. Takakura and colleagues [21] treated 18 patients who had ankle osteoarthritis with low tibial osteotomy for varus tilt of the tibial plafond. Fifteen of 18 patients achieved good results, with decreased medial joint space narrowing. The study authors noted that correction of the tabiotalar angle and varus deformity decreased the need for lateral ankle ligament reconstruction. Myerson and Miller [24] and Haddad and colleagues [25] have also described the association between the cavovarus foot and heel varus with chronic ankle instability. Scranton and colleagues [13] developed a malleolar index to measure and document a posteriorly positioned fibula. They hypothesized that this anatomic variant created a more vulnerable open ankle mortise that predisposed these patients to chronic ankle instability. In fact, 52.1% of their unstable ankle population had a more posteriorly positioned fibula. They also found 65% of the 23 patients in the CAT scan study with a malleolar index greater than +15°

had a history of an ankle sprain. They documented that patients who have unstable ankles have a 3.37 times greater incidence of ankle joint spurs or loose bodies related to anterior tibial impingement or to degenerative arthritis than normal volunteers [13]. Reick and colleagues [22] showed that higher grades of ankle osteoarthritis were 5 to 10 times more prevalent in 209 patients who had chronic ankle instability.

Harrington [19] reported 36 patients who had chronic lateral ankle instability with radiographic evidence of ankle osteoarthritis. He did not specifically state whether a cavovarus foot alignment was present, but did note inversion of the hindfoot and radiographic findings of medial joint space narrowing and varus talar tilt. Fortin and colleagues [15] looked at 10 patients who had 13 idiopathic cavovarus feet with chronic lateral ankle instability, all of which had varying degrees of osteoarthritis. Ten of these patients had varus tilting of the talus with intermediate to advanced osteoarthritis of the ankle joint. Six patients had advanced osteoarthritis underwent ankle arthrodesis. Four patients who had mild or intermediate changes were treated with a lateral displacement calcaneal osteotomy, with or without first metatarsal dorsiflexion osteotomy and lateral ankle ligament reconstruction. All patients had improvement of the varus ankle alignment, and 12 of 13 feet had neutral to slight valgus heel alignment. All patients had improvement of functional scores and resolution of symptoms of ankle instability. The study authors felt that their series of patients represented the natural history of long-standing untreated ankle instability and cavovarus foot deformity. They proposed that cavovarus foot deformity in patients who have chronic lateral ankle instability may have important implications relating to the development of ankle arthritis secondary to increased contact stresses, and also that correction of the cavovarus deformity may help to normalize forces acting across the ankle, aiding in the effectiveness of a lateral ankle ligament reconstruction [15].

Operative procedures for flexible deformity: soft-tissue realignment procedures

Isolated reconstruction of the lateral ankle ligaments for instability in the cavovarus foot will often fail if the contributing foot deformity is not addressed at the time of operative treatment [7,15]. Recurrent sprains of the ankle or subtalar joint can be treated with tightening of the lateral ankle ligaments, with or without augmentation. Most authors describe a Bröstrom or anatomic repair of the lateral ankle ligaments, combined with a lateral displacement type of calcaneal osteotomy, with or without a first-metatarsal dorsiflexion osteotomy and gastrocnemius lengthening [15]. This may be combined with ankle arthroscopy to debride anterior impingement or degenerative ankle osteophytes [13,15]. A Strayer gastrocnemius recession or a modified Vulpius lengthening can be done through a medial incision, cutting through the gastrocnemius tendon alone, and occasionally through the soleus fascia if more lengthening is required [7,8,26,27].

For a flexible, plantarflexed, first ray deformity with peroneal overdrive, a peroneus longus to peroneus brevis tendon transfer is done at the peroneal tubercle, with tubercle resection, allowing the tendon to gap 1.5 cm [7]. The distal peroneus longus stump is transferred to the brevis tendon in a side-to-side tenodesis. This is done to avoid the formation of a dorsal bunion. Associated peroneal tendon pathology, such as a peroneal tendon tear with or without dislocating peroneal tendons, may require repair of the tendon tear with tightening of the superior retinaculum. A shallow peroneal fibular groove may need to deepened as well to prevent recurrent dislocation. In some cases, a lateral displacement calcaneal osteotomy may also be warranted with severe hindfoot varus, in order to help prevent recurrent dislocation and decrease peroneal stress or strain.

Operative treatment for flexible deformity: metatarsal and calcaneal osteotomies

If the patient continues to experience pain related to cavovarus foot and ankle deformity despite the appropriate treatment, then surgical reconstructive procedures are performed. The goals of operative treatment of the cavovarus foot and ankle are to reduce deformity and instability in order to create a stable plantigrade foot and allow more normal joint contact pressures during gait. It is preferable to preserve motion to decrease stiffness in order to prevent or slow down the onset of degenerative joint changes whenever possible. To accomplish these goals, both metatarsal and calcaneal osteotomies have been combined with soft-tissue procedures, to avoid or prolong the need for arthrodesis in the flexible cavovarus foot [28,29].

Swanson and colleagues [30] described the use of dorsal closing wedge metatarsal osteotomies with plantar fascial release for the treatment of the cavovarus foot. Watanabe [31] described first through fifth metatarsal osteotomies combined with plantar fasciotomies and other various procedures. A chevron osteotomy of the first metatarsal was used for increased stability of the first ray, and oblique or dorsally based closing wedge osteotomies were performed for the lesser metatarsals without fixation. Many calcaneal osteotomies have been described in the orthopedic literature for the treatment of the cavovarus foot and ankle. Dwyer [32] described a laterally based closing wedge osteotomy with division of the plantar fascia for the treatment of the cavovarus foot. Samilson and Dillin [33] described a crescenteric calcaneal osteotomy for hindfoot-driven cavus.

Gould [34] employed the use of Dwyer's calcaneal osteotomy with proximal metatarsal base osteotomies for patients who had cavovarus feet and Charcot-Marie-Tooth disease. He reported that at 4.5 years all patients had increased peroneal muscle strength, with continued or increased foot flexibility. Sammarco and Taylor [28,29] combined a lateral superior sliding calcaneal osteotomy with dorsolateral closing wedge proximal metatarsal osteotomies in 21 feet for a painful rigid neuropathic cavovarus foot. At an average follow-up of 49.8 months, an 89% good-to-excellent outcome using the American Orthopaedic Foot and Ankle Society (AOFAS) score was obtained. Sixteen of the 21 patients maintained or improved their foot motion. Radiographs confirmed correction or improvement of the cavovarus foot deformity with a 13% reduction in longitudinal arch height, as well as varus forefoot and heel deformity. Fortin and colleagues [15] treated 5 idiopathic cavovarus feet in 4 patients who had chronic ankle instability with mild to intermediate ankle osteoarthritis with a combination of osteotomies and soft-tissue realignment procedures. Two patients (3 feet) had mild degenerative changes with anterior ankle osteophytes without talar tilt. Two patients (2 feet) had intermediate degenerative changes with medial joint space narrowing and varus tilt of the talus. In 2 feet this involved first metatarsal dorsiflexion osteotomy, lateral displacement calcaneal osteotomy, and lateral ankle ligament reconstruction. One patient underwent bilateral ankle anterior osteophyte removal, lateral ankle ligament reconstruction, and calcaneal osteotomy. All patients had improvement of the varus alignment of the ankle and hindfoot with a neutral to slight valgus heel. All patients had improvement of functional ankle scores with resolution of instability.

These clinical studies demonstrate that there is no one procedure that by itself will allow correction of a cavovarus foot and ankle deformity. Multiple procedures are required for reduction of a multiplanar deformity through realignment procedures of the ankle, hindfoot, midfoot, and forefoot. In patients who have a relatively flexible deformity, this is best accomplished through the combination of calcaneal and metatarsal osteotomies to preserve joint motion even in the presence of osteoarthritis (Fig. 1). Also, in most patients the bony procedures need to be combined with soft-tissue realignment procedures, such as lateral ankle ligament reconstruction, gastrocnemius lengthening, plantar fascial release, or peroneus longus tenotomy and transfer. These procedures act to restore a more normal alignment, and therefore mechanical axis, to the foot and ankle attempting to distribute joint forces and loads more evenly. This is important to help prevent osteoarthritis, relieve symptoms of existing arthrosis, and delay its progression while preserving motion and delaying or preventing the need for arthrodesis.

Surgical technique for metatarsal osteotomy

A first metatarsal dorsiflexion osteotomy is performed in most patients. The need for osteotomy of the second through fifth metatarsals is determined clinically based on the individual contribution of each metatarsal to the cavus deformity. The first metatarsal osteotomy can be done as a chevron type of osteotomy or a dorsal closing wedge ostoetomy of the first metatarsal base. Beals and Manoli [8] described a V-type chevron osteotomy of the first metatarsal just 1 cm distal to the tarsometatarsal joint fixed with

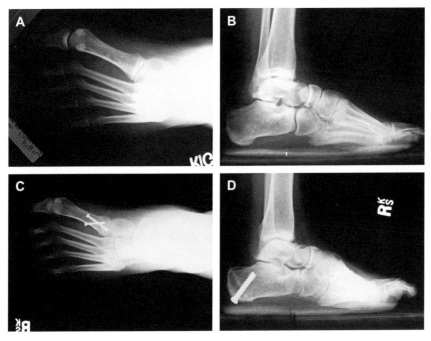

Fig. 1. *A* and *B* are preoperative radiographs of a flexible cavovarus foot in a 17-year-old who has Charcot-Marie-Tooth disease with chronic lateral ankle instability and symptoms of lateral column overload. *C* and *D* are postoperative radiographs of the same patient after superolateral displacement calcaneal osteotomy with first metatarsal dorsiflexion osteotomy, combined with lateral ankle ligament reconstruction and gastrocnemius lengthening.

a 4.0 mm screw. Care should be taken to notch or countersink the cortex of the metatarsal in order to avoid breakage of the bony cortical bridge. Sammarco and Taylor [28,29] describe a dorsolateral closing wedge osteotomy of the first metatatarsal for additional correction, with the same osteotomies of the second through fifth metatarsal bases as necessary for correction. The dorsolateral closing wedge osteotomies of the first and second metatarsals are performed through a longitudinal incision placed just distal to the first tarsometatarsal joint. The third, fourth, and fifth metatarsal bases can be exposed with a longitudinal incision over the fourth metatarsal. A subperiosteal dissection is performed at the junction of the base and the metaphyses, and a dorsolateral-based closing wedge osteotomy is performed 1 cm distal to the tarsometatarsal joint. The proximal limb of the osteotomy is made perpendicular to the long axis of the metatarsal and the distal limb oblique to this cut to produce a dorsolateral-based wedge, the dimensions of which will vary from patient to patient depending on the correction necessary. Once the wedge is removed, a dorsolateral pressure on the forefoot to the midfoot will close the osteotomy. The osteotomies are fixed with one or two crossed 0.045 mm or 0.062 mm Kirschner wires that are bent, cut, and buried beneath the skin. The first metatarsal osteotomy can also be fixed with two crossed 3.0 mm or 3.5 mm cannulated screws, depending on the size of the metatarsal and the bone quality of the patient. These procedures are almost always performed in conjunction with a calcaneal osteotomy with various soft-tissue procedures, and require a short leg, non-weight–bearing cast for about 8 weeks to heal in the majority of patients.

Surgical technique for lateral displacement calcaneal osteotomy

The patient is positioned supine with a bump under the ipsalateral hip. Surgery is performed under general anesthesia using a thigh tourniquet. A 4-cm oblique incision is made laterally over the calcaneus, anterior to the Achilles tendon insertion, from the posterior superior tuberosity to the anteroinferior tuberosity. A subperiosteal dissection is made in line with the incision, and a transverse osteotomy is performed from lateral to medial across both cortices, perpendicular to the long axis of the calcaneus, with a large oscillating saw. The posterior fragment is then translated laterally 5 to 10 mm until the heel is in physiologic valgus if possible. Sammarco and colleagues [28,29], describe a dorsolateral displacement calcaneal osteotomy for maximal correction, which involves translating the proximal fragment 1 cm dorsal as well as lateral. If more correction is needed, then a laterally based closing wedge osteotomy can be performed [35]. A second saw cut can be made just distal to the first cut, angling slightly proximal to remove a small laterally based wedge. The wedge is removed and closed down on the lateral cortex. The osteotomy is then fixed with one or two 6.5 mm, partially threaded, cannulated screws from posterior to anterior under fluoroscopic guidance. Subperiosteal stripping of the soft-tissue attachments on the plantar posterior fragment may be necessary to allow adequate translation of the osteotomy. Sammarco and colleagues [28,29] also describe a small medial incision on the non-weight–bearing portion of the midfoot to sharply divide the plantar fascia, in order to decrease arch height if necessary. As discussed previously, this procedure is usually combined with a gastrocnemius lengthening as well. These procedures require a short leg, non-weight–bearing cast for 8 weeks in most patients to heal; if not longer in a neuropathic patient who has poor-quality bone.

Operative treatment for rigid varus deformity: hindfoot arthrodesis

A triple arthrodesis of the hindfoot combines fusion of the subtalar joint with fusion of the talonavicular and calcaneocuboid joints. The purpose of a triple arthrodesis is to restore and provide a plantigrade stable foot. This is usually done for rigid cavovarus deformity in order to decrease pain and improve function and stability by realigning the hindfoot joints. This also aids in realigning the ankle joint and treating or preventing recurrent skin breakdown and stress fractures along the lateral column. Levitt and colleagues [36] examined 30 cavovarus feet with different neuromuscular disorders, and discovered that eventual triple arthrodesis was required in almost all of the patients. Recent studies have demonstrated its efficacy for pain relief and overall patient satisfaction. Beischer and colleagues [37] and Pell and colleagues [38] have shown patient satisfaction rates of 90% or greater more than 5 years post-surgery; however, one must be careful with the position of arthrodesis and its effect on the remaining joints in the foot and the mechanical axis of the ankle. In fact, long-term results have shown deterioration to 47% poor results at an average of 21 years post-surgery, with up to 40% of patients complaining of continued pain [39]. Others have reported recurrence of preoperative deformity in 9% to 20% of patients, particularly those who have neuromuscular disorders as the etiology of their cavovarus deformity [40–43]. Nonunion and pseudoarthrosis of the arthrodesis can occur up to 6% to 33% of the time, and can be a cause of continued pain [42–44]. This risk is significantly higher in the neuromuscular patient population [34,36,39,45]. The use of bone graft can greatly reduce the risk of nonunion by establishing an extra-articular arthrodesis in the sinus tarsi [46]. Pell and colleagues [38] reported only a 2% nonunion rate with the use of adjuvant bone graft for triple arthrodesis. Fortin and Walling [47] confirmed these findings, with only a 3% nonunion rate using similar operative techniques.

Even when done properly and for the appropriate reasons, the triple arthodesis is done at the expense of subtalar and transverse tarsal joint motion [48]. The loss of motion in the hindfoot also results in altered biomechanics to the remaining articulations of the ipsalateral limb, decreased power, and distorted gait patterns that may result in functional loss. This results from the loss of shock absorption offered by intact joints and the increased stress placed on the surrounding joints by the loss of hindfoot mobility. One third of patients will walk with a limp, with most patients experiencing difficulty with walking on uneven terrain [37,48]. Also, a long-term study of 44-year follow-up found that 68% of patients walked with an assistive device [44]. Though the surgery offers significant relief of preoperative pain, most patients will experience some continued hindfoot pain [48]. Patients may also complain of knees and hip pain after triple arthrodesis [44,48].

To avoid an in situ arthrodesis for severe cavovarus deformity, as well as incomplete reduction of the deformity and malunion, modifications of a more standard triple arthrodesis technique may be required to restore a more anatomic alignment to the foot and ankle [35,49]. It should be remembered that like the treatment of the flexible cavovarus foot and ankle, the treatment of the rigid cavovarus deformity should be augmented with osteotomies of the calcaneus and first metatarsal, along with gastrocnemius lengthening when necessary to provide maximal correction (Fig. 2). Pell and colleagues [38] found a significant correlation between the correction of

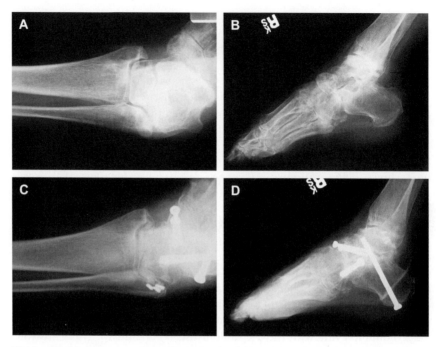

Fig. 2. *A* and *B* are preoperative radiographs of a rigid cavovarus foot deformity after a stroke. The radiographs are non-weight–bearing; the patient was unable to bear weight on the extremity because of the painful deformity. *C* and *D* are postoperative radiographs after triple arthrodesis with superolateral displacement calcaneal osteotomy and first metatarsal dorsiflexion osteotomy. This patient also required an open Achilles lengthening, as well as an extensive posteromedial release of the soft tissues.

deformity and postoperative patient satisfaction. To date, several techniques have been described in the literature specifically for the treatment of a rigid cavovarus deformity. Haddad and colleagues [25] described revision triple arthrodesis using extended laterally based wedge resections of the hindfoot joints, with or without calcaneal osteotomy, in the treatment of patients who have a malunion of a triple arthrodesis. Siffert and colleagues [50] have described a "beak" triple arthrodesis for the treatment of severe cavus foot deformity. This used similar wedge resection of the subtalar joint, combined with a dorsally based closing wedge osteotomy of the transverse tarsal joints. Manoli and Graham [7] remind us that in long-standing rigid cavovarus deformities, reducing the heel into slight physiologic valgus in the presence of a plantarflexed first ray will only increase its plantarflexion. If this is not recognized and treated with a first metatarsal dorsiflexion osteotomy, the ankle joint will fall into compensatory varus.

Therefore, these clinical studies demonstrate that a well-done, modified triple arthrodesis with the appropriate concomitant osteotomies and soft-tissue realignment procedures can satisfactorily reduce rigid cavovarus deformity and pain. The key is to recognize and address as many of the components of the cavovarus deformity as possible at the time of surgical treatment.

Surgical technique for hindfoot arthrodesis

Because most physicians are familiar with the standard technique, this author focuses on the modified triple arthrodesis technique for the cavovarus hindfoot [35,49]. A standard two-incision approach, one dorsomedial and one lateral, is used for a standard or modified triple arthrodesis for the cavovarus foot. Both the Siffert [50] beakand Haddad and colleagues [25] modified triple arthodesis use similar techniques and principles of closing wedge hindfoot joint resection in conjunction with hindfoot arthrodesis to reduce cavovarus deformity. In the beak technique the soft-tissue attachments to the talar head are left intact. A laterally based wedge resection of the subtalar joint is performed with a saw or osteotome. A dorsally based wedge resection of the calcaneocuboid joint is then similarly performed. The plantar portion of the talar head is removed, leaving the superior half of the talar head intact to preserve blood supply. A dorsally based wedge excision of the proximal navicular is then performed, allowing translation of the navicular inferiorly and the calcaneus laterally [50]. In the modified triple arthrodesis technique, a laterally based closing wedge resection of the subtalar joint is also used, along with a laterally based closing wedge osteotomy of the transverse tarsal joints [25,35,49]. This could be made biplanar with a dorsal wedge component if necessary for maximal correction. If additional correction is needed for hindfoot varus, then a lateral displacement calcaneal osteotomy, with or without superior displacement, can be employed to further reduce hindfoot deformity [24,35]. Also a modified laterally based Dwyer closing wedge calcaneal osteotomy could also be used in adjunct [24,35]. Once the desired correction is obtained, then the subtalar joint athrodesis site, as well as the calcaneal osteotomy when done, can be fixed using 6.5 mm or 7.3 mm cannulated screws. The tranverse tarsal joint arthrodesis sites can be fixed with 4.5 mm cannulated screws. These surgeries require a short leg, non-weight–bearing cast for 2 to 3 months to heal.

Operative treatment of the rigid varus ankle: ankle arthrodesis versus replacement

As previously discussed, many, if not all, patients who have a cavovarus foot and ankle deformity will develop degenerative osteoarthritis of the ankle joint over time [7,13,15,18]. Early to moderate ankle osteoarthritis can be addressed without arthrodesis with the use of calcaneal and metatarsal osteotomies combined with gastrocnemius lengthening and debridement of osteophytes, with lateral ankle ligament reconstruction when appropriate [7,19,28,30]. If significant varus malalignment of the distal tibia or joint is also present, this can be addressed with a supramalleolar osteotomy of the distal tibia to unload the more arthritic portion of the joint and provide a more anatomic mechanical axis to the ankle itself, redistributing joint contact forces and loads [3,20,21,51]. Most patients who have end-stage varus osteoarthritis of the ankle with a rigid cavovarus foot, however, can only be realigned and treated with a combination of ankle or modified hindfoot arthrodesis to provide a stable plantigrade foot (Fig. 3). Fortin and colleagues [15] studied six patients who had eight cavovarus foot and ankles with end-stage osteoarthritis of the ankle joint, characterized by varus tilt of the talus and joint space obliteration. These patients underwent ankle arthrodesis, with three feet also undergoing simultaneous dorsiflexion osteotomy of the first metatarsal for a supple hindfoot deformity. There were no nonunions and the follow-up ranged from 12 months to 62 months. All but one patient had a neutral to slight valgus heel alignment, with the remaining patient having residual heel varus. All patients had improvement of functional ankle scores with resolution of instability, and would have the procedure done again. For patients who have severe rigid varus ankle and hindfoot deformity with end-stage osteoarthritis, a pantalar arthrodesis is effective to provide a stable plantigrade foot (Fig. 4); however, this

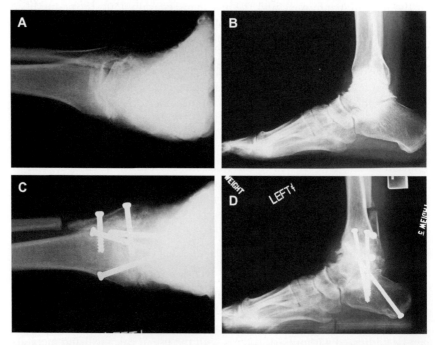

Fig. 3. *A* and *B* are preoperative radiographs of a rigid idiopathic cavovarus foot and ankle with end-stage varus ankle osteoarthritis secondary to chronic lateral ankle instability. *C* and *D* are postoperative radiographs after a tibiotalocalcaneal arthrodesis with superolateral displacement calcaneal osteotomy and gastrocnemius lengthening.

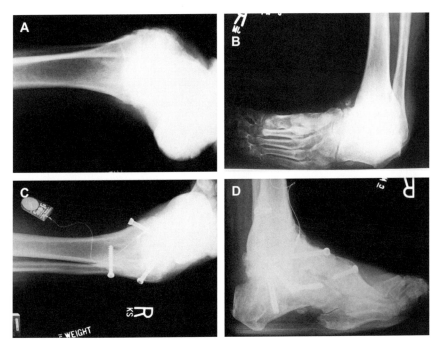

Fig. 4. *A* and *B* are preoperative radiographs of a 65-year-old man who had Charcot-Marie-Tooth disease and a severe, rigid cavovarus foot and ankle, with end-stage varus ankle osteoarthritis and recurrent stress fractures of the lateral metatarsals from walking on his lateral midfoot. *C* and *D* are postoperative radiographs after some hardware removal from a pantalar arthrodesis with superolateral displacement calcaneal osteotomy, combined with a first metatarsal dorsiflexion osteotomy and open Achilles tendon lengthening.

procedure may also require the same modifications as the author's ankle or triple athrodesis to accomplish this goal, such as a lateral displacement calcaneal osteotomy, first metatarsal or lesser metatarsal osteotomy, and gastrocnemius lengthening.

In some cases the varus osteoarthritic ankle can be treated with a total ankle arthroplasty, combined with hindfoot arthrodesis or realignment procedures that address the underlying cavovarus deformity [24,52]. The prostheses are minimally constrained, and can often tip into varus postoperatively if the underlying cavovarus deformity is not addressed. Though a lateral displacement calcaneal osteotomy for flexible hindfoot varus can be done at the time of total ankle arthroplasty, hindfoot arthrodeses are usually performed as staged procedures for rigid deformities [24]. If only an isolated subtalar joint arthrodesis is needed, with or without calcaneal osteotomy, this can sometimes be done concomitantly with the replacement (Fig. 5) [24]; however, this could be problematic with talar vascular necrosis from soft-tissue stripping. This author concurs with Myerson and Miller [24] that an arthrodesis should be a staged procedure when done with a total

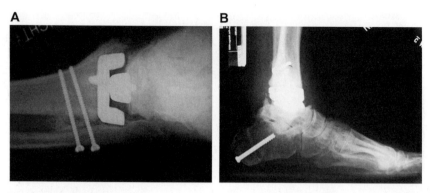

Fig. 5. *A* and *B* are postoperative radiographs of a 55-year-old patient who had an idiopathic flexible cavovarus foot with chronic ankle instability, resulting in varus ankle osteoarthritis. He underwent total ankle replacement and superolateral displacement calcaneal ostoetotmy, combined with lateral ankle ligament reconstruction and gastrocnemius lengthening.

ankle replacement, with 4 months or longer in between. The prolonged casting required for healing of a hindfoot arthrodesis my result in less than satisfactory motion of the ankle joint when done simultaneously with arthroplasty. Chronic lateral ankle instability often accompanies hindfoot or tibiotalar varus deformity, which can be problematic for prosthetic stability even if soft- tissue rebalancing is performed [7,15,20]. When necessary, a lateral ankle ligament reconstruction can be performed at the time of total ankle arthroplasty [24,52]. Typically, for a varus hindfoot with an unstable varus osteoarthritic ankle, the deltoid ligament is tight and needs to be released for complete medial and lateral soft-tissue rebalancing, along with the lateral ankle ligament reconstruction [24,52]. All patients should be counseled that if the total ankle replacement fails and cannot be revised, then an ankle arthrodesis would be performed.

Surgical technique for ankle arthrodesis

There are many different techniques described for ankle arthrodesis. The best approach takes into account the apex of the main deformity, the cause of the injury, any pre-existing soft-tissue damage, and the need for additional procedures at the time of surgery. An anterior approach can be used when the talus has been displaced laterally or medially under the tibia in the frontal plane, or when a pre-existing surgical incision is already there [52]. The patient is supine with a bump underneath the ipsalateral hip. A standard anterior incision is made medial to the anterior tibial tendon sheath and lateral to the neurovascular bundle and extensor hallucis longus tendon. It is placed about 3 inches proximal to the ankle joint extending distally to the talar neck. A subperiosteal dissection is performed along with an arthrotomy of the ankle joint. The tubercle of Chaput is excised with an osteotome through a vertical cut made parallel to the fossa holding the fibula. Removal of the tubercle allows debridement of the notch and close approximation of the fibula to both the tibia and the lateral talus for fixation. All cartilage and osteophytes are scraped from the talar dome, the medial and lateral gutters of the joint, and the distal tibial plafond. This is usually performed with one quarter inch curved and straight osteotomes and small curved and straight curettes. Hard subchondral bone is then perforated diffusely in the joint surface to allow bleeding subchondral bone, with a 2.0 mm or a 2.5 mm drill bit to facilitate arthrodesis. Care should be taken to maintain the general anatomic configuration or shape of the joint in order to allow bone-on-bone contact for arthrodesis and to prevent further shortening of the limb. The ankle joint is then positioned into neutral plantarflexion/dorsiflexion and slight valgus, with the talus positioned back in the mortise to bring the mechanical axis of the joint just anterior to the plafond. Screw fixation is then performed.

The inside-out technique is then used to place the first screw from the posterior malleolus to the anterior neck or head of the talus [52]. The foot is positioned into plantarflexion, and a 4.5 mm drill is used to make a retrograde gliding hole for a 6.5 mm, partially threaded lag screw, with a 16 mm thread length, aiming 4 to 6 cm above the joint and lateral to the Achilles. A 4.0 mm suction tip is then placed through the hole to the skin, and a small skin incision is made at that site. A long 3.5 mm drill bit is then inserted into the suction tip from the posterior incision, guiding the drill bit into the joint. The ankle is then into the position of fusion and the drill bit is advanced into the talus. The drill hole in the tibia is measured and then 30 mm is added to it to accommodate the talus. The suction tip is then used in the same fashion to bring the screw to the appropriate hole in the distal tibia for insertion. The ankle is then aligned into the position of arthrodesis, and the screw is advanced. Then at least three more 6.5 mm screws are placed using the same drill bits and lag screw technique. The first is place from the medial malleolus to the midbody of the talus at about a 45° angle. The second of these screws is from the midlateral malleolus and aimed transversely toward the posterior talar body. The third screw is placed from the anterolateral distal tibia to the posterior talar body. A shear-strain–relieving bone graft is then placed into the anterior side of the joint to augment arthrodesis. Bone graft should also be placed between the tibia and the fibula where compressed by screw fixation. The skin is then closed in the usual fashion and a short leg splint applied. These patients are made non-weight–bearing in a short leg cast for 8 weeks after surgery, though some patients may require up to 3 to 4 months of healing time, depending on bony quality and other risk factors.

A lateral approach is indicated when the foot is translated forward because of an old anterior pilon fracture or when lateral hardware is present and requires removal [52]. It is also the approach of choice when a pantalar or tibiotalocalcaneal fusion will be performed to minimize soft-tissue stripping. The patient is positioned the same way as for the anterior approach. A straight lateral incision is made over the anterior border of the fibula or through the old fibular incision, from the tip to about 6 to 7 cm proximally. The fibula is then osteotomized obliquely, and the inner or medial third is excised to expose bleeding subchondral bone. The fibula is then allowed to roll back posteriorly on its soft-tissue attachments. The joint is then prepared in the same fashion as for the anterior approach. The screws can then be placed in a similar way, except that the posterior-to-anterior screw can be placed under direct visualization. In the final step, the fibula is replaced against the distal tibia and talus and is fixed in this position with two 3.5 mm or 4.5 mm compression screws. One screw is placed into the tibia and the other into the talus. The same postoperative regimen can be applied with this approach. The current cannulated 6.5 mm screw systems can be used for these ankle arthrodesis techniques, and are very useful with an unstable malaligned ankle joint as well as being more user friendly when assistance is limited or unavailable.

Operative treatment for varus tibial deformity: supramalleolar osteotomy

Significant malalignment of the distal tibia alters the mechanical axis of the ankle joint and causes altered load distribution and ankle joint mechanics [53,54]. Over time this has been shown to cause increased joint stress, pain, and cartilage wear, resulting in degenerative osteoarthritis. Currently, no specific guidelines exist for the acceptable limits of angulation in the distal tibia to prevent these complications from occurring, though several studies have found that distal tibial angulation of 10° or less in the frontal or sagittal plane is consistent with normal ankle function without symptoms of pain [55,56]. Biomechanical cadaveric studies have demonstrated decreased ankle joint contact surface area up to 40% secondary to malalignment [53,54]. In addition, Tarr and colleagues [53] showed that distal tibia deformity greatly altered ankle joint contact area, shape, and location. Ting and colleagues [54] had similar findings of altered joint contact with distal tibia deformity. More importantly, they found that the subtalar joint acts as a torque transmitter when compensating for coronal plane deformities, and is important in maintaining tibiotalar alignment. This may come into play in fixed cavovarus deformities with a stiff subtalar joint or hindfoot, which would increase tibiotalar contact forces above that normally seen from isolated angular deformities of the tibia, thereby increasing the chance of degenerative arthritis. In fact, several studies have documented the presence of hindfoot pain, stiffness, and osteoarthritis after distal tibial fractures with malalignment [57,58].

The supramalleolar osteotomy has been described previously in the pediatric orthopedic literature for the treatment of congenital or acquired equinocavovarus deformities, from residual clubfoot or post-polio syndrome [59,60]. It has also been used in the pediatric population for the treatment of growth disturbance and resultant angular deformity after physeal injury [61]. In the adult population it has been used in the correction of angular deformity of the distal tibia, with or without resultant osteoarthritic change of the ankle joint [3,20,21,51,62]. The angular deformity may result from a malunion of a distal tibial metaphyseal or ankle pilon fracture or a congenital malalignment of the limb or extremity (Fig. 6). Two previous studies have been done on the use of the supramalleolar osteotomy for symptomatic post-traumatic varus malalignment of the distal tibia associated with osteoarthritis [62,63]. They found that it was effective to realign the ankle joint to a neutral position and reduce the symptoms of pain and the progression of pre-existing ankle joint osteoarthritis. One group of researchers, Takakura and colleagues [21], also has published a study using the supramalleolar osteotomy for idiopathic varus osteoarthritis of the ankle joint. They used an opening medially based wedge osteotomy of the distal tibia to redistribute the joint stress and contact force to the more normal or less arthritic portion of the ankle joint. This successfully decreased patients' pain and increased their function while slowing down or halting progression of the pre-existing arthritis of the joint.

More recently Stamatis and colleagues [3] performed supramalleolar osteotomies for the correction of distal tibial malalignment of at least 10° for pain, with or without radiographic osteoarthritic changes. Two patients had a varus malunion of the distal tibia after distal tibia or ankle pilon fracture, with or without osteoarthritis. Four patients had a varus ankle deformity with osteoarthritis. The rest had valgus deformity of the distal tibia. On all patients the center of rotation and angulation (CORA) was determined to plan for corrective osteotomy. The CORA was determined to be located at the intersection of two lines that represent the mechanical axes of the

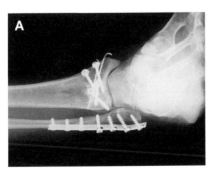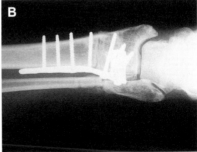

Fig. 6. *A* is a preoperative radiograph of a patient who had a varus deformity of the distal tibia after an open distal tibiofibular fracture with early post-traumatic osteoarthritis of the ankle. *B* is a postoperative radiograph after a laterally based closing wedge osteotomy of the tibia and fibula. The decision for the lateral closing wedge osteotomy versus a medial opening osteotomy was based on the patient's previous open medial wound and local skin grafting done in that area.

proximal and distal fragments of the fractures. All patients who had varus deformities were treated with a medial based opening wedge osteotomy. Several patients had additional procedures done at the time of surgery for maximal correction of their deformities, including one lateral displacement biplanar calcaneal osteotomy. All underwent Achilles tendon lengthening and three underwent arthroscopic ankle debridement of degenerative osteophytes. Average time to healing was 14 weeks, and the average follow-up was 33.6 months. At final follow-up, all patients had significantly decreased ankle pain, with no progression in their arthritic changes on radiographs. Only one of these patients developed a delayed union of the osteotomy that required reoperation and bone grafting.

These clinical studies have shown that the distal tibia supramalleolar osteotomy is a reliable operative treatment for realignment of distal tibia angular deformity, post-traumatic and otherwise, and its resultant osteoarthritic changes of the ankle joint. It helps relieve both the symptoms of arthritis pain by restoring a more normal mechanical axis, and slows down the progression of pre-existing osteoarthritis. This is an important alternative to delay or try to prevent the need for ankle arthodesis for the varus malaligned ankle.

Operative technique for supramalleolar osteotomy

Varus deformities can be treated with either a medial opening wedge or a lateral closing wedge supramalleolar osteotomy [3,20,21,51,62]. A medial based opening wedge osteotomy is preferable to prevent shortening of the extremity and a resultant limb length discrepancy, which can often already be present from a post-traumatic deformity or osteoarthritis [3]; however, a laterally based, closing wedge osteotomy of the distal tibia and fibula can also be used with great success. This technique is particularly useful after varus malunion of an open distal tibia or ankle pilon fracture, where the medial soft-tissue envelope is poor or damaged. If the osteotomy is being done to correct post-traumatic deformity, it should be located at the level of the CORA [3]. In cases of isolated angular deformity, the CORA is at the apex of the deformity. In cases of very distal tibia deformities, the CORA is at the level of the ankle joint. It is important to determine the CORA because a closing or opening wedge osteotomy done at the CORA will lead to complete realignment of the ankle. If done proximal or distal to the CORA, the osteotomy may cause a translational deformity of the distal fragment, shifting the mechanical axis of the joint [3]. In patients such as those who have a varus ankle without fracture in which the CORA is at the level of the ankle joint, medial translation of the distal fragment is necessary to restore and maintain a normal mechanical axis of the ankle joint.

In distal tibial deformities in which the CORA is at the level of the ankle joint without significant angular deformity of the more proximal tibia, the osteotomy should be performed 4 to 5 cm proximal to the medial malleolar tip [3].

A short oblique fibular osteotomy is performed first, through a small lateral incision at the same level of the planned tibial cut. No fixation of the fibular osteotomy is required. A medial longitudinal incision is made over the site of the planned tibial cut, and a subperiosteal dissection is performed in line with the planned cut. A horizontal osteotomy is made with a large oscillating saw to the distal tibia, preserving the lateral cortex as a hinge to aid in stability. The osteotomy is then gently distracted with a lamina spreader under fluoroscopic guidance, until the desired correction or neutral joint alignment is achieved. The space is then filled with an appropriately shaped bone graft such as iliac crest or tibial tubercle autograft with allograft supplementation when necessary, though this procedure can be performed using allograft iliac crest graft with supplementation, such as with platelet gel. The osteotomy is then fixed using a distal tibial periarticular plate and screw system. The patient is then made non-weight–bearing in a short leg cast for 3 to 4 months until healed.

Discussion

As this article demonstrates, the cavovarus foot and ankle is a complex deformity with many different etiologies. Each cavovarus foot and ankle is different and needs to be properly assessed to determine the appropriate operative management for each patient. There are only general guidelines for operative management, and no specific treatment algorithm has been described to date. The clinical studies demonstrate that there is no one procedure that by itself will allow correction of a cavovarus foot and ankle deformity. Multiple procedures are required for reduction of a multiplanar deformity through realignment procedures of the ankle, hindfoot, midfoot, and forefoot.

In patients who have a flexible deformity based on the Coleman block test, this is best accomplished through the combination of calcaneal and metatarsal osteotomies to preserve joint motion, even in the presence of osteoarthritis. Also, in most patients, the bony procedures need to be combined with soft-tissue realignment procedures, such as lateral ankle ligament reconstruction, gastrocnemius lengthening, plantar fascial release, or peroneus longus tenotomy and transfer. These procedures act to restore a more normal alignment, and therefore more normal mechanical axis, to the foot and ankle attempting to distribute joint forces and loads more evenly. This is important to help prevent osteoarthritis, relieve symptoms of existing arthrosis, and delay its progression while preserving motion and delaying or preventing the need for arthrodesis.

In a smaller patient population, a total ankle replacement may be possible to avoid the need for ankle arthrodesis; however, this needs to be combined with underlying hindfoot realignment procedures such as calcaneal osteotomy, subtalar or triple arthrodesis, and lateral ankle ligament reconstruction for soft- tissue rebalancing. In the case of isolated varus tibia deformity, post-traumatic or congenital, a supramalleolar osteotomy of the distal tibia and fibulas can be used to obtain a neutral joint. This acts to distribute loads more evenly across the ankle and offload any existing osteoarthritis, relieving pain and helping to prevent progression of the osteoarthritis.

In cases of rigid and nonreducible deformity, selective arthrodesis should be undertaken. The rigid cavovarus foot and ankle can be addressed using a modified triple arthrodesis, an ankle arthrodesis, a tibiotalocalcaneal arthrodesis, or pantalar arthrodesis. The number of joints selected for fusion should be individualized for each patient according to rigidity and amount of osteoarthritis present. Care must always be taken to avoid in situ arthrodesis, and to use the discussed techniques to reduce the foot and ankle into as neutral a position as possible for functional gait and more normalized joint contact pressures or loads. This can be done by a modified resection of the joint to reduce deformity, as well as by the addition of calcaneal and metatarsal osteotomies.

In summary, our goals for the cavovarus foot and ankle reconstruction are to preserve motion whenever possible and to maintain or impart stability, while realigning foot and ankle joints into as anatomic a position as possible, in order to restore a more normal mechanical axis to the extremity and redistribute joint pressure or load more evenly.

References

[1] McCluskey WP, Lovell WW, Cummings RJ. The cavovarus foot deformity: etiology and management. Clin Orthop 1989;247:27–37.

[2] Manoli A 2nd, Smith DG, Hansen ST Jr. Scarred muscle excision for the treatment of established ischemic contracture of the lower extremity. Clin Orthop 1993;292:309–14.

[3] Stamatis ED, Cooper PS, Myerson MS. Supramalleolar osteotomy for the treatment of distal tibial angular deformities and arthritis of the ankle joint. Foot Ankle Int 2003;24: 754–64.

[4] Steucker RD, Bennett JT. Tarsal coalition presenting as a pes cavo-varus deformity; report of three cases and review of the literature. Foot Ankle 1993;14:540–4.

[5] Holmes JR, Hansen ST Jr. Foot and ankle manifestations of Charcot-Marie-Tooth disease. Foot Ankle Int 1993;14:476–86.

[6] Mosca VS. The cavus foot. J Pediatr Orthop 2001;21:423–4.

[7] Manoli A 2nd, Graham B. The subtle cavus foot "the underpronator," a review. Foot Ankle Int 2005;26:256.

[8] Beals TC, Manoli A 2nd. Late varus instability with equines deformity. J Foot Ankle Surg 1988;4:77–81.

[9] Digiovanni CW, Kuo R, Tejwani N, et al. Isolated gastrocnemius tightness. J Bone Joint Surg Am 1990;72:962–70.

[10] Coleman SS, Chestnut WJ. A simple test for hindfoot flexibility in the cavovarus foot. Clin Orthop 1977;123:60–2.

[11] Ledoux WR, Shofer JB, Ahroni JH, et al. Biomechanical differences among pes cavus, neutrally aligned, and pes planus feet in subjects with diabetes. Foot Ankle Int 2003;24: 845–50.

[12] Chadha H, Pomeroy GC, Manoli A 2nd. Radiologic signs of unilateral pes planus. Foot Ankle Int 1997;18:603–4.

[13] Scranton PE Jr, McDermott JE, Rogers JV. The relationship between chronic ankle instability and variations in mortise anatomy and impingement spurs. Foot Ankle Int 2000;21:657–64.

[14] Saltzman CL, El-Koury GY. The hindfoot alignment view. Foot Ankle Int 1995;16:572–6.

[15] Fortin PT, Guettler JH, Manoli A 2nd. Idiopathic cavovarus foot and lateral ankle instability: recognition and treatment implications relating to ankle arthritis. Foot Ankle Int 2002;23:1031–7.

[16] Steffensmeier SJ, Saltzman CL, Berbaum KS, et al. Effects of medial and lateral displacement calcaneal osteotomies on tibiotalar joint contact stresses. J Orthop Res 1996; 14:980–5.

[17] Buckwalter JA, Saltzman CL. Ankle osteoarthritis: distinctive characteristics. Instr Course Lect 1999;48:233–42.

[18] Ramsey PL, Hamilton W. Changes in tibiotalar area of contact caused by lateral talar shift. J Bone Joint Surg Am 1976;58:356–7.

[19] Harrington KD. Degenerative arthritis of the ankle secondary to long–standing lateral instability. J Bone Joint Surg Am 1979;61:354–61.

[20] Sugimoto K, Samoto N, Takakura Y, et al. Varus tilt of the tibial plafond as a factor in chronic ligament instability of the ankle. Foot Ankle Int 1997;18:402–5.

[21] Takakura Y, Tanaka Y, Kumai T, et al. Low tibial osteotomy for osteoarthritis of the ankle. J bone Joint Surg 1995;77B:50–4.

[22] Rieck B, Reiser M, Bernet P. Posttraumatic arthrosis of the upper ankle joint in chronic insufficiency of the fibular ligament. Orthopade 1986;6:466–71.

[23] Colville MR. Surgical treatment of the unstable ankle. J Acad Orthop Surg 1998;6:368–77.

[24] Myerson MS, Miller SD. Salvage after complications of total ankle arthroplasty. Foot Ankle Clin 2002;7:191–206.

[25] Haddad SI, Myerson M, Pell RF, et al. Clinical and radiographic outcome of revision surgery for failed triple arthrodesis. Foot Ankle Int 1997;18:489–99.

[26] Pinney SJ, Hansen ST, Sangeorzan BJ. The effect on ankle dorsiflexion of gastrocnemius recession. Foot Ankle Int 2002;23:26–9.

[27] Saraph V, Zwick EB, Uitz W, et al. The Baumann procedure for fixed flexion contracture of the gastrocsoleus in cerebral palsy. J Bone Joint Surg 2000;82B:535–40.

[28] Sammarco GJ, Taylor R. Combined calcaneal and metatarsal osteotomies for the treatment of the cavus foot. Foot Ankle Clin 2001;6:533–43.

[29] Sammarco GJ, Taylor R. Cavovarus foot treated with combined calcaneus and metatarsal osteotomies. Foot Ankle Int 2001;22:19–30.

[30] Swanson AB, Browne HS, Coleman JD. The cavus foot—concepts of production and treatment by metatarsal osteotomy. J Bone Joint Surg Am 1966;48:1019.

[31] Watanabe RS. Metatarsal osteotomy for the cavus foot. Clin Orthop 1990;252:217–30.

[32] Dwyer FC. The present status of the problem of pes cavus. Clin Orthop 1975;106:254–75.

[33] Samilson RL, Dillin W. Cavus, cavovarus, and calcaneocavus: an update. Clin Orthop 1983; 177:125–32.

[34] Gould N. Surgery in advanced Charcot-Marie-Tooth disease. Foot Ankle Int 1984;4: 267–73.

[35] Sullivan R, Aranow M. Different faces of the triple arthrodesis. Foot Ankle Clin 2002;7: 95–106.

[36] Levitt RL, Canale ST, Cooke AJ Jr, et al. The role of foot surgery in progressive neuromuscular disorders in children. J Bone Joint Surg Am 1973;55:1396–410.

[37] Beischer AD, Bridsky JW, Pollo FE, et al. Functional outcome and gait analysis after triple arthrodesis. Foot Ankle Int 1999;20:545–53.

[38] Pell RF, Myerson MS, Schon LC. Clinical outcome after primary triple arthrodesis. J Bone Joint Surg Am 2000;82:47–57.

[39] Wetmore RS, Drennan JC. Long-term results of triple arthrodesis in Charcot-Marie-Tooth disease. J Bone Joint Surg Am 1989;71:417–22.

[40] Figgie MP, O'Malley MJ, Ranawat C, et al. Triple arthrodesis in rheumatoid arthritis. Clin Orthop 1993;292:250–4.

[41] Haritidis JH, Kirkos JM, Provellegios SM, et al. Long-term results of triple arthrodesis: 42 cases followed for 25 years. Foot Ankle Int 1994;15:548–51.

[42] Sangeorzan BJ, Smith D, Veith R, et al. Triple arthrodesis using internal fixation in the treatment of adult foot disorders. Clin Orthop 1993;294:299–307.

[43] Wukich DK, Bowen JR. A long-term study of triple arthrodesis for correction of pes cavovarus in Charot-Marie-Tooth disease. J Pediatr Orthop 1989;9:433–7.

[44] Saltzman CL, Fehrle MJ, Cooper RR, et al. Triple arthrodesis: twenty-five and forty-four-year average follow-up of the same patients. J Bone Joint Surg Am 1999;81:1391–402.

[45] Mann DC, Hsu JD. Triple arthrodesis in the treatment of fixed cavovarus deformity in adolescent patients with Charcot-Marie-Tooth disease. Foot Ankle Int 1992;13:1–6.

[46] Williams PF, Menelaus MB. Triple arthrodesis by inlay grafting—a method suitable for the underformed or valgus foot. J Bone Joint Surg Br 1977;59:333–6.

[47] Fortin PT, Walling AK. Triple arthrodesis. Clin Orthop 1999;365:91–9.

[48] Gellman H, Lenihan M, Halikis N, et al. Selective tarsal arthrodesis: an in vitro anaylsis of the effect on foot motion. Foot Ankle Int 1987;8:127–33.

[49] Raiken S. Failure of triple arthrodesis. Foot Ankle Clin 2007;7:121–34.

[50] Siffert RS, Forster RI, Nachamie B. "Beak" triple arthrodesis for correction of severe cavus foot deformity. Clin Orthop 1966;45:101.

[51] Cheng Y, Chang J, Hsu C, et al. Lower tibial osteotomy for osteoarthritis of the ankle. Kaohsiung Journal Medical Society 1994;10:430–7.

[52] Hansen ST. Ankle arthrodesis. In: Hurley R, Seigafuse SL, Marino-Vasquez D, editors. Functional reconstruction of the foot and ankle. Philadelphia: Lippincott Williams and Wilkins; 2000. p. 283–90.

[53] Tarr RR, Resnick CT, Wagner KS, et al. Changes in tibiotalar joint contact areas following experimentially induced tibial angular deformities. Clin Orthop 1985;199:72–80.

[54] Ting AJ, Tarr RR, Sarmiento A, et al. The role of subtalar motion and ankle contact pressure changes from angular deformities of the tibia. Foot Ankle 1987;7:290–9.

[55] Merchant TC, Dietz FR. Long-term follow-up after fractures of the tibial and fibular shafts. J Bone Joint Surg Am 1989;71:599–606.

[56] Kretensen KD, Kiaer T, Bilcher J. No arthrosis of the ankle 20 years after malaligned tibial-shaft fracture. Acta Orthop Scand 1989;60:208–9.

[57] Merriam WF, Porter KM. Hindfoot disability after a tibial shaft fracture treated by internal fixation. J Bone Joint Surg Br 1983;65:326–8.

[58] McMaster M. Disability of the hindfoot after fracture of the tibial shaft. J Bone Joint Surg Br 1976;58:90–3.

[59] McNicol D, Leong JC, Hsu LC. Supramalleolar derotation ostoetomy for lateral tibial torsion and associated equinovarus deformity of the foot. J Bone Joint Surg Am 1983;65:166–70.

[60] Napiontek M, Nazar J. Tibial osteotomy as a salvage procedure in the treatment of congenital talipes equinovarus. J Pediatr Orthop 1994;14:763–7.

[61] Scheffer MM, Peterson HA. Opening wedge osteotomy for angular deformities of long bones in children. J Bone Joint Surg Am 1994;76:325–34.

[62] Takakura Y, takaoka T, Tanaka Y, et al. Results of opening-wedge osteotomy for the treatment of a post-traumatic deformity of the ankle. J Bone Joint surg Am 1998;80:213–8.

[63] Graehl PM, Hersh MR, Heckman JD. Supramalleolar osteotomy for the treatment of symptomatic tibial malunion. J Orthop Trauma 1987;1:281–92.

ELSEVIER
SAUNDERS

Foot Ankle Clin N Am
12 (2007) 177–195

FOOT AND
ANKLE CLINICS

Ankle Instability and Impingement

Anthony D. Watson, MD

*Greater Pittsburgh Orthopaedic Associates, 5820 Centre Avenue,
Pittsburgh, PA 15206, USA*

Ankle sprains are extremely common injuries and chronic disability is rare. Two common causes of chronic disability after ankle sprain are instability and impingement. Each may take several forms, and the typical contributing factors include failure to seek treatment, undertreatment, recurrent injuries, and youth. Treatment of instability often responds to rehabilitation but may require surgery. Symptomatic, disabling impingement usually requires surgery.

Ankle instability

Anatomy and pathomechanics of ankle injury

Ankle stability depends on static stability conferred by the bony architecture of the ankle joint. The ankle can be thought of as a mobile mortise and tenon joint, also known as a tongue and groove joint, wherein the talus is the tenon that fits into the mortise, or groove, composed of the distal tibia and fibula. The talus is wider anteriorly than posteriorly; thus, the talus is not as well contained by the mortise when plantarflexed as when dorsiflexed. The dorsal surface of the talus has a slight longitudinal groove that corresponds to a longitudinal ridge on the tibial plafond. The ridge and groove help confer transverse plane stability of the tibiotalar joint.

The ankle ligaments provide supplemental stability to the ankle and also contribute to hindfoot stability. The lateral and medial ligaments primarily stabilize against inversion and eversion, respectively, but also provide rotatory stability that is often not considered by treating physicians. Table 1 and Figs. 1 and 2 detail the anatomy and functions of the primary ankle ligaments.

Important considerations regarding the functional anatomy of the ankle ligaments include the role of the anterior talofibular ligament (ATFL) in

E-mail address: watsonad@verizon.net

1083-7515/07/$ - see front matter © 2007 Elsevier Inc. All rights reserved.
doi:10.1016/j.fcl.2006.12.007

WATSON

Table 1
Comparison of the major stabilizing ligaments of the ankle

Ligament	Origin	Insertion	Tightest in	Stabilizes
Anterior talofibular	Anterior margin of distal fibula	Lateral aspect of talar neck	Plantarflexion	Inversion in plantarflexion
Calcaneofibular	Medial aspect of tip of fibula	Lateral wall of calcaneus, posterior to longitudinal axis of fibula	Dorsiflexion	Inversion in dorsiflexion
Anterior inferior tibiofibular	Anterior margin of fibula at syndesmosis	Anterior distal tibia at syndesmosis	Dorsiflexion	External rotation of talus in dorsiflexion
Deltoid	Medial malleolus	Talus, calcaneus, spring ligament, navicular	Different bands tighten in various positions of dorsiflexion/ plantarflexion	Eversion in any position of dorsiflexion/ plantarflexion

controlling anteromedial rotatory stability, the insertion of the calcaneofibular ligament (CFL) posterior to the longitudinal axis of the fibula (see Fig. 1), and the different roles of the multiple bands of the deltoid ligament (see Fig. 2). The ATFL courses obliquely from posterolateral to anteromedial with respect to the tibiotalar joint. It thus resists internal rotation of the talus and not just anterior translation. The CFL courses posteriorly from its origin on the tip of the fibula to insert on the calcaneus posterior to the fibula. As a result, it is coplanar with the fibula in 10° to 20° of dorsiflexion—an

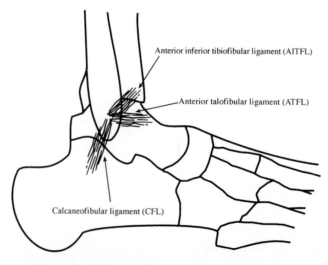

Fig. 1. Lateral ankle detailing the major stabilizing ligaments.

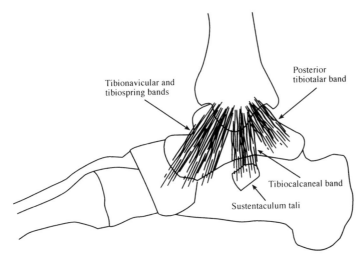

Fig. 2. Medial ankle detailing the major consistent bands of the deltoid ligament.

important consideration when performing physical examination or reconstructing the CFL. Finally, the deltoid ligament can be composed of as many as six bands divided into two layers. The most consistent bands are the deep posterior tibiotalar, the tibiospring, and the tibionavicular [1]. The deep posterior tibiotalar band is the medial equivalent of the CFL and the tibiospring and tibionavicular bands are the medial equivalent of the ATFL.

The medial and lateral talocalcaneal interosseous ligaments are capsular thickenings that contribute to eversion and inversion stability, respectively, of the subtalar joint. The role of the cervical ligament is less well defined but is largely believed to be a secondary inversion stabilizer of the subtalar joint [2]. Its strain increases when the calcaneofibular ligament is insufficient [3].

The musculotendinous units that cross the ankle joint provide dynamic stability to the ankle and hindfoot. The most important of these are the peroneal tendons and the posterior tibialis tendon, which stabilize against inversion and eversion, respectively. Chronic lateral or medial instability can cause overuse injury, such as tendonitis or rupture, to the peroneal tendons or posterior tibialis tendon, respectively.

The classic ankle sprain occurs with inversion of the plantarflexed ankle when the forefoot is bearing weight. Maximum elongation and tension of the ATFL occurs in plantarflexion. Forced inversion while in plantarflexion can increase ligament stress and strain beyond the yield point (stretch or partial tear) or even the ultimate failure strain (complete tear) (Fig. 3). The force may be sufficient to also injure the CFL. More commonly, failure of the ATFL causes rebound dorsiflexion of the ankle as the heel comes back into contact with the ground. Continued inversion force with the ankle

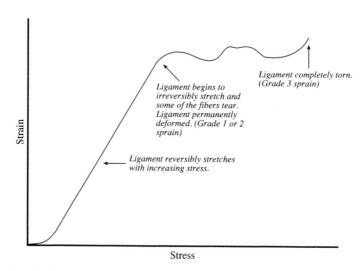

Fig. 3. Hypothetical stress–strain curve depicting ligament behavior. No permanent deformation occurs with stress in the straight line segment of the curve. Injury begins to occur where the curve transitions from straight line to the curved line. Complete failure of the ligament occurs at the rightmost point of the curve.

in neutral or dorsiflexion leads to yield point or ultimate failure strain of the CFL.

The high ankle sprain, an anterior inferior tibiofibular ligament (AITFL) injury caused by internal rotation of the leg on a planted foot that is fully plantigrade, has received increased attention in the last several years. Because the talus is wider anteriorly, there is little rotatory motion possible in the transverse plane. As the leg rotates interiorly on the talus, the talus wedges the syndesmosis apart. The Maisonneuve fracture, comprising deltoid ligament rupture, AITFL rupture, and proximal fibula fracture, is a higher-energy form of the high ankle sprain.

Pathophysiology

Chronic ankle instability and ankle impingement result from inadequate and inappropriate healing after ligamentous injury. Chronic ankle instability results when the injured ligaments do not regain the mechanical integrity necessary to stabilize the ankle against physiologic stress. Varus tibial plafond alignment, varus hindfoot alignment, or a posterior fibular position can predispose to chronic ankle instability [4–7]. Peroneal or posterior tibialis tendonitis can develop from overuse of the dynamic stabilizers that attempt to stabilize the unstable ankle. Another cause of ankle pain with instability is increased stress on the intact ligaments. This finding is especially common with medial instability [1].

Anterior soft tissue ankle impingement can be attributable to hypertrophic fibrosis of the injured ligament that in turn is entrapped in the ankle joint with motion. This impingement typically affects the ATFL, AITFL, or the anterior tibiotalar or tibionavicular bands of the deltoid ligament (Fig. 4) [8–12]. Posterior soft tissue impingement can be caused by hypertrophic fibrosis of a previously injured posterior tibiotalar band of the deltoid ligament, transverse tibiofibular ligament, or posterior capsule inflammation from repetitive stress [11–13].

Anterior bony impingement typically results from chronic ankle instability leading to posttraumatic arthrosis with osteophyte formation [14]. The osteophytes are likely attributable to progressive degenerative changes rather than capsular traction [15]. Posterior bony impingement can be attributable to an unstable os trigonum, fracture, or nonunion of the trigonal (posterolateral) process of the talus, or repetitive compression of either the os trigonum or trigonal process of the talus [13].

Patient evaluation

Box 1 details the differential diagnoses to consider when evaluating a patient for instability or impingement. Fig. 5 presents a diagnostic algorithm.

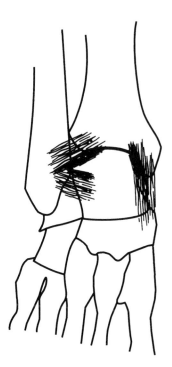

Fig. 4. Typical areas of anterior impingement occur along the inferior margin of the AITFL, the superior margin of the ATFL, and the medial margin of the anterior tibiotalar and tibionavicular bands of the deltoid ligament.

**Box 1. Comparison of the differential diagnosis of ankle
instability and impingement**

Instability
Dynamic
    Inadequate rehabilitation
    Neuromuscular deficit
Reflex inhibition
    Pain
    Tarsal coalition
    Ankle tendonitis
Mechanical
    Lateral
    Medial
    Syndesmotic

Impingement
Anterior
    Soft tissue
    Bony
Posterior
    Posteromedial soft tissue
    Os trigonum
    Trigonal process
    Capsular impingement

History

"My ankle gives out on me" is a common complaint of many people who have any number of ankle abnormalities after one or more sprains. It is imperative to determine whether or not they have mechanical instability, reflex inhibition because of pain from any cause, or dynamic instability. Mechanical and dynamic instability are better evaluated with physical examination, whereas reflex inhibition can be diagnosed largely by history.

Pain with giving-way typically occurs after the episode when there is mechanical instability, whereas pain before a giving-way episode implies reflex inhibition. Giving-way attributable to mechanical instability is more frequent on uneven ground or in running sports when the involved leg is the outside leg while turning or running in a curved pattern. Deceleration maneuvers in sports are also frequent causes. Descending stairs or a slope can cause giving-way because these activities require weight bearing on the forefoot with the ankle in plantarflexion.

Any activity that positions the ankle in one of its extremes of motion causes impingement pain. Leaning forward on a planted foot, ascending

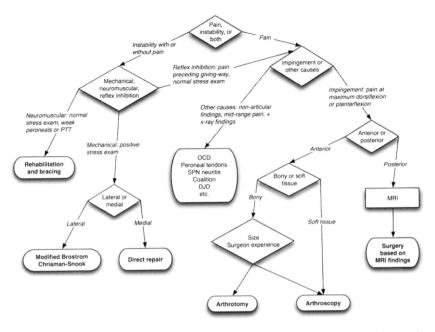

Fig. 5. Diagnostic algorithm for patients presenting with ankle instability with or without pain.

stairs or a slope, and squatting can all cause anterior impingement pain. Classically, posterior impingement has been considered an occupational disease of ballet; however, jumping and explosive athletic activity, such as leaving a starting block in a track sprint or leaving the offensive or defensive line on the snap of the football, can cause posterior impingement pain. Pain associated with the impingement can cause reflex inhibition giving-way of the ankle.

Physical examination

After thorough vascular and sensory examination, it is important to assess the standing alignment of the ankle and hindfoot. Varus of either the ankle or hindfoot predisposes the ankle to instability and peroneal tendon pathology. Hindfoot valgus can predispose to medial instability and posterior tibialis tendon dysfunction. Plantarflexion of the talus associated with planovalgus deformity can predispose to posterior impingement. Ligamentous lateral ankle instability is mechanically unlikely with pes planovalgus alignment, but tarsal coalition with subjective instability may be present. Hindfoot valgus on weight bearing that can be corrected by the patient by painless activation of the posterior tibialis suggests medial instability [1].

Active and passive range of motion should each be assessed. Limited passive hindfoot range of motion suggests tarsal coalition. Limited active eversion suggests inadequate rehabilitation of the peroneal musculotendinous units. Pain at extreme passive dorsiflexion implies anterior impingement. Painful limitation of passive dorsiflexion with a block preventing expected ankle dorsiflexion suggests bony anterior impingement. Pain at extreme passive plantarflexion implies posterior impingement. Tenderness over the anterior ankle, posterolateral ankle between the peroneal tendons and Achilles tendon, and posteromedial ankle increases suspicion of anterior, posterolateral, and posteromedial impingement, respectively.

It is possible to reproduce anterior impingement pain by palpating the anterolateral ankle in plantarflexion, then dorsiflexing the ankle while maintaining pressure with the examiner's digit over the anterolateral ankle. An increase in pain is 95% sensitive and 88% specific for anterior soft tissue impingement [16].

Accurate and reliable stability testing requires attention to anatomic and technical detail. When possible, compare the stress examination to the contralateral ankle given the wide population variability of bony anatomy and ligamentous laxity.

Remember that the ATFL courses anteromedially from the distal fibula. Furthermore, the tibionavicular band of the deltoid ligament courses from posterior to anterior. Isolated testing of the ATFL therefore requires anteromedial rotatory drawer stress of the plantarflexed ankle (Fig. 6) to reduce the possibility of a false negative stability examination caused by an intact tibionavicular band of the deltoid that could limit anterior excursion of the talus relative to the distal tibia. Because the CFL does not contribute to stability in plantarflexion, anteromedial rotatory drawer should be done with the ankle plantarflexed to isolate the ATFL.

The CFL stabilizes the ankle and subtalar joint against inversion in the dorsiflexed ankle; therefore, stress examination of the CFL consists of inverting the hindfoot with the ankle dorsiflexed. Subtalar instability may

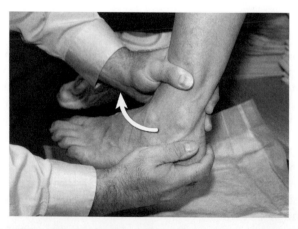

Fig. 6. Anteromedial rotatory drawer maneuver to test the ATFL in isolation. The arrow depicts the force applied to the foot while holding the leg superior to the ankle.

be appreciated by applying adduction force to the forefoot while maintaining inversion and internal rotation stress to the heel while the ankle is in 10° of dorsiflexion [17]. Medial shift of the calcaneus and opening of the talocalcaneal joint compose a positive test.

Pain over the AITFL with external rotation of the dorsiflexed foot and ankle implies distal tibiofibular syndesmosis instability. The squeeze test, wherein the fibula and tibia are squeezed together in the midleg, also reproduces pain at the distal tibiofibular syndesmosis when unstable. Unlike tests of the ATFL and CFL, no appreciable motion occurs with stability testing of the distal tibiofibular syndesmosis, and therefore pain indicates a positive test [18].

Deltoid ligament instability can be difficult to assess because of its multiple bands and broad origin and insertions. It is unlikely that the ankle will open medially with eversion stress; instead, pain localized to the band of the deltoid being tested implies instability. The posterior bands of the deltoid (superficial posterior tibiotalar and deep posterior tibiotalar) are stressed by everting the dorsiflexed ankle, the middle band (tibiocalcaneal) by everting the neutral ankle, and the anterior bands (tibiospring, tibionavicular, and deep anterior tibiotalar) by anterolateral rotatory drawer of the plantarflexed ankle.

Ankle strength, especially the peroneals and the posterior tibialis, should be critically evaluated. Lateral ankle instability may be associated with peroneal tendonitis, rupture, or subluxation.

Diagnostic testing

Radiographs should include anteroposterior (AP), lateral, and oblique views. Whenever possible, these should be obtained in a weight-bearing position to assess syndesmotic alignment, angulatory malalignment of the tibial plafond, and mortise congruency with load. The ankle is typically plantarflexed when non–weight-bearing radiographs are obtained, which positions the narrower portion of the talus in the mortise and can lead to a false positive interpretation of tibiotalar incongruity. A weight-bearing lateral radiograph of the ankle with the patient leaning far forward over the planted foot can demonstrate anterior bony impingement. Additional anterior bony detail can be obtained with an oblique radiograph as described by Tol and colleagues [19]. A non–weight-bearing lateral radiograph of the maximally plantarflexed ankle can demonstrate posterior bony impingement by the posterior process of the talus or an os trigonum. Osteochondral lesions may accompany ankle instability or ankle impingement.

Various manual and mechanical methods have been described to obtain stress radiographs. Meta-analysis has determined that stress radiography by any method is not sufficiently rigorous to be useful, however [20]. Diagnosis and treatment planning for ankle instability therefore depend on clinical parameters.

Obtaining reliable, reproducible MRI of the ankle ligaments and intra-articular soft tissue pathology remains challenging. Often, little more than evidence of prior injury to an ankle ligament is all that can reliably be determined. Normal ligaments typically have a striated appearance, whereas the appearance of an injured ligament can range from a homogenous appearance without striations to greater than normal diameter to severe thinning or loss of continuity.

MRI is useful to rule out causes of ankle pain other than instability or impingement, and it is useful when associated pathology, such as an osteochondral lesion or peroneal tendon rupture, is suspected.

Clinical findings are often sufficient for the diagnosis and treatment of anterior soft tissue impingement. If MRI is necessary to help confirm the diagnosis, however, MR arthrography or contrast-enhanced, fat-suppressed, three-dimensional (3D), fast-gradient-recalled acquisition in the steady state with radio-frequency-spoiling (CE 3D-FSPGR) MRI is necessary to achieve adequate sensitivity, specificity, positive predictive value, negative predictive value, and accuracy [21–23]. CE 3D-FSPGR has the advantage that invasive arthrography is not necessary. Plain MRI lacks accuracy [24] unless an effusion is present [25]. MRI arthrography findings diagnostic of anteromedial or anterolateral soft tissue impingement include thickening or nodularity of the soft tissues in the region of the AITFL and ATFL, and limited distention of the capsule by contrast in either the anterolateral or anteromedial recess (Fig. 7) [22,23]. Findings on CE 3D-FSPGR MRI that diagnose soft tissue impingement include thickening and enhancement of the soft tissues in the region of the AITFL and ATFL or anterior deltoid [21].

Unenhanced MRI is useful in the diagnostic evaluation and treatment planning of posterior impingement. There is often a soft tissue component

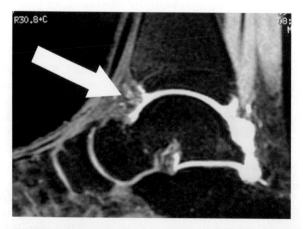

Fig. 7. MRI arthrogram of the ankle depicting anterior soft tissue impingement. The arrow points to an anterior soft tissue impingement lesion occupying the anterior recess of the ankle, which, when normal, should fill the way the posterior ankle has filled in this MRI.

to the pain that cannot be imaged with plain radiographs, and physical examination does not have enough resolution to discern between the anatomic structures that could be responsible for the pain [26]. Furthermore, multiple sources of pain may coexist, such as flexor hallucis longus (FHL) tendonitis with os trigonum pain in dancers [13,26,27].

Intra-articular injection of local anesthetic helps to differentiate impingement from extra-articular causes of anterior ankle pain, such as superficial peroneal nerve traction neuritis, extensor tendonitis, and postinjury pain syndrome. Injection of local anesthetic posterior to the ankle is not as specific for differentiating posterior ankle pain diagnoses given the infiltration of several different tissues.

Treatment

Indications

Disabling mechanical instability after adequate rehabilitation of the dynamic ankle stabilizers (peroneals and posterior tibialis) is an indication for surgical treatment. The patient should be advised that pain may or may not be resolved and they should not have the expectation that surgery is for pain relief. The patient should also understand that some range of motion will likely be lost to gain stability.

Likewise, disabling impingement pain that does not improve with appropriate nonoperative measures, such as an in-shoe heel lift for anterior impingement and activity restriction for anterior or posterior impingement, is an indication for surgical treatment. Anterior soft tissue impingement can be easily managed arthroscopically, whereas bony impingement may require arthrotomy to achieve adequate decompression. Surgical treatment of posterior impingement typically requires an open approach to the ankle.

Ankle ligament reconstruction

The two basic forms of ankle ligament reconstruction are anatomic and nonanatomic procedures. The most common anatomic technique is the modified Brostrom procedure, which consists of reefing of the ATFL and CFL and then reinforcing the repair by proximally advancing the inferior extensor retinaculum. This procedure minimizes the loss of range of motion [28].

The most commonly reported nonanatomic techniques are the Chrisman-Snook reconstruction and the Evans reconstruction. Both techniques use the peroneus brevis tendon to reconstruct the lateral ankle ligaments. The advantage of these procedures is the use of healthy tissue, but range of motion and eversion strength are compromised [29–31]. The results of nonanatomic reconstruction are not as good as anatomic reconstruction with regard to persistent and recurrent instability, limitation of motion, and altered gait kinematics [28,32–36]. Recurrent instability after Evans tenodesis may be because of not stabilizing the subtalar joint [2].

Direct repair, possibly including suture anchors, is performed to reconstruct deltoid ligament instability [1]. A tendon graft procedure has been described for reconstructing syndesmosis instability [37].

Modified Brostrom procedure

A curvilinear incision is made along the anterior border of the distal fibula and extends distally and posteriorly along the tip of the fibula. Full-thickness tissue flaps are elevated anteriorly to expose the ATFL and inferiorly to expose the peroneal tendons and the calcaneal tuberosity. It is important to expose the calcaneus posterior to the fibula because the CFL attachment is relatively posterior on the calcaneus. The peroneal tendons must be retracted from their sheath to expose the underlying CFL.

The ATFL and CFL are inspected and if adequate tissue extends from the fibula, a capsulotomy is made along the same line as the skin incision so that the residual ATFL and CFL are transected. Occasionally, the most attenuated portion of either ligament is at the fibular attachment. When this is the case, the attenuated tissue is excised and periosteum is elevated from the underlying fibula to create flaps for later repair to the residual ATFL and CFL.

Redundant and unhealthy tissue is débrided. Nonabsorbable, braided 2-0 sutures are placed so that the transected ligaments and capsule are advanced and shortened, but are not tied until all have been placed. The ankle is dorsiflexed and everted while applying a posterior drawer and the sutures placed in the ATFL tightened and tied. The ankle is then gently plantarflexed and everted and the sutures placed in the CFL are tightened and tied. The remaining capsular sutures are then tightened and tied.

The inferior extensor retinaculum is then mobilized by blunt dissection, advanced proximally to the area of reconstruction, and repaired to the reconstruction with absorbable, braided 3-0 suture. The wound is closed in layers, and the ankle is immobilized in a posterior splint with the foot and ankle in eversion and resting flexion.

A removable walker boot is applied 2 weeks after surgery and used for 6 weeks for a total of 8 weeks of immobilization. The patient must be non–weight bearing for 4 weeks. Active, nonresistive ankle and hindfoot exercises are initiated by the patient 2 weeks after surgery and physical therapy is begun 6 to 8 weeks after surgery. The earliest athletic activity may resume is 3 months after surgery and depends on the patient's ability to maintain single-limb balance with the eyes closed for at least 30 seconds, perform 30 side-to-side hops on the involved leg, and hop up a single step on the involved leg.

Chrisman-Snook procedure

The skin incision begins 3 cm proximal to the tip of the fibula, continues parallel to the peroneal tendons, and extends to the base of the fifth metatarsal. The sheaths enclosing the peroneus brevis are all divided. A full-thickness flap is elevated anteriorly to expose the anterior ankle as far as the lateral neck of the talus. The peroneal tendons are elevated from the underlying calcaneus inferior to the fibula.

The peroneus brevis tendon is divided longitudinally starting at its insertion into the base of the fifth metatarsal and extending proximally. The half of the peroneal tendon with less muscular attachment is then transected as far proximally as possible and a nonabsorbable braided 2-0 suture placed in the stump using a whip stitch or grasping stitch technique.

Classically, the tendon graft is passed through drill tunnels in the distal fibula and calcaneus. Techniques using suture anchors or interference screws have been described recently [38,39]. The technique for anchoring the tendon graft to bone is not as important as the placement of the tendon graft anchor points.

A tunnel is made in the distal fibula with a drill and curette. The tunnel connects the fibular origin of the ATFL and the fibular origin of the CFL. The tendon is first anchored to the lateral neck of the talus with the ankle dorsiflexed and everted while applying a posterior drawer. The tendon is then passed through the tunnel in the distal fibula. While maintaining ankle dorsiflexion, eversion, and posterior drawer, tension is applied to the transferred tendon and it is repaired to the soft tissues at the anterior fibula with 2-0 nonabsorbable braided suture and then to the soft tissues at the posterior fibula. The remaining tendon is then anchored to the calcaneus with the ankle plantarflexed and everted (Fig. 8). To ensure correct placement of the calcaneal anchor point, it is helpful to first mark the point, which is 1 cm posterior to the longitudinal axis of the fibula with the ankle in neutral position.

The wound is closed in layers, and the ankle is immobilized in a posterior splint with the foot and ankle in eversion and resting flexion. A removable walker boot is applied 2 weeks after surgery and used for 6 weeks for a total of 8 weeks of immobilization. The patient must be non–weight bearing for 4 weeks. Active, nonresistive ankle and hindfoot exercises are initiated by the patient 2 weeks after surgery and physical therapy is begun 6 to 8 weeks after surgery. The earliest athletic activity may resume is 3 months after surgery and depends on the patient's ability to maintain single-limb balance with the eyes closed for at least 30 seconds, perform 30 side-to-side hops on the involved leg, and hop up a single step on the involved leg.

Deltoid ligament repair

Repair is performed through a direct approach through the sheath of the posterior tibialis tendon. The attenuated portion of the deltoid ligament should be transected, débrided, shortened, and then repaired while

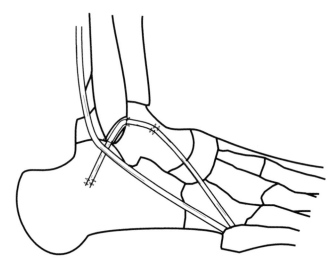

Fig. 8. Chrisman-Snook procedure wherein one half of the peroneus brevis is anchored to the lateral aspect of the talar neck, then passed through a tunnel in the distal fibula where it is anchored at the entrance and exit of the tunnel, and then passed to the lateral calcaneus where it is anchored approximately 1 cm posterior to the posterior aspect of the fibula.

maintaining the ankle and hindfoot in inversion. Suture anchors may be necessary to facilitate repair. The ankle should be in plantarflexion for repair of the posterior tibiotalar band, neutral for the tibiocalcaneal band, and in dorsiflexion with posterior drawer for the tibiospring and tibionavicular bands. Wound closure and postoperative care is the same as for lateral ankle ligament reconstruction.

Ankle impingement

Arthroscopic treatment of anterior ankle soft tissue impingement is highly successful and the results are reliably reproducible [10,15,21,40–44]. Bony impingement can also be successfully treated arthroscopically because the osteophytes are intra-articular and not capsular [45]. Excellent to good results are less frequent than after arthroscopic treatment of anterior soft tissue impingement, and the results are worse with higher grades of osteoarthritis [15,46]. Open treatment may be necessary depending on the size of the osteophytes [47] and the surgeon's experience with arthroscopic technique.

Arthroscopic anterior ankle decompression

Soft tissue impingement lesions arising from the AITFL, ATFL, or deltoid are usually amenable to arthroscopic treatment. The standard anteromedial and anterolateral portals are used and the hypertrophic tissue débrided with a power shaver until normal ligamentous tissue is identified.

Hypertrophic tissue is typically dull white and amorphous in appearance, whereas normal ligamentous tissue is shiny, organized, and made up of parallel bundles of fibers (Fig. 9).

The portals should be closed with nylon suture and a removable walker boot applied over a dressing in the operating room. Weight bearing and range-of-motion exercises should start in a week if the incisions are healing uneventfully.

Arthroscopic decompression of bony impingement can be technically difficult, as is the case with arthroscopic subacromial decompression of the shoulder, and thus depends on the surgeon's experience. A power burr is used to gradually remove osteophytes from the anterior margin of the tibia until the articular cartilage is seen in cross-section. The talar osteophytes are removed until slight saucerization has occurred. It is imperative not to remove excessive bone from the talus because a fracture may develop through cortical bone that has been compromised.

Significant bony impingement is more amenable to open decompression. An anteromedial incision and arthrotomy is usually sufficient but an anterolateral incision may also be necessary. The tibial osteophytes are typically located laterally and the talar osteophytes are typically located medially [48]. The osteophytes can be easily removed with an osteotome; bone is gradually removed from the distal tibia until the articular cartilage margin is identified. Bone from the talar neck osteophytes is gradually removed until the normal contour of the talar neck is identified. There often is capsular and synovial hypertrophy that contributes to the impingement, which must also be débrided.

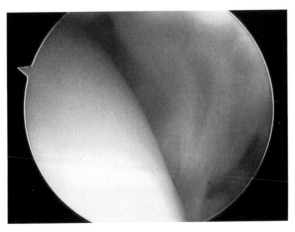

Fig. 9. Arthroscopic view of an anterior soft tissue impingement lesion. The view is looking anterolateral from a medial portal. The talus occupies the left half of the picture, and the soft tissue lesion arising from the inferior margin of the AITFL occupies the right half of the picture.

The wounds are closed in layers and a removable walker boot applied over a dressing in the operating room. Weight bearing and range-of-motion exercises should start in a week if the incisions are healing uneventfully.

Posterior ankle impingement

There is significant radiographic variability in patients who have posterior ankle impingement symptoms; therefore, the MRI findings are important to preoperative planning. Most posterior impingement pathology can be approached surgically from posterolateral. A posteromedial approach is necessary for débridement of a posteromedial soft tissue impingement lesion; otherwise, the posterolateral approach is more useful [12].

Components of posterior ankle impingement that may show increased signal intensity on T2-weighted MRI and thus require excision or débridement include the os trigonum, the trigonal process, the posterior ankle or subtalar joint capsule and synovium, the soft tissues posterior to the ankle and subtalar joint, the posterior tibiotalar band of the deltoid ligament, and the transverse posterior tibiofibular ligament [11–13,49]. Stenosing tenosynovitis of the FHL may be present also and require decompression of the FHL sheath [13].

For a posterolateral approach, the patient is positioned in lateral decubitus and the interval between the Achilles tendon and peroneal tendons is developed. Full-thickness tissue flaps are essential, but care must be taken to identify and protect the sural nerve.

The soft tissues posterior to the ankle are often edematous and should be excised. The trigonal process of the talus or os trigonum can be palpated and visualized in the interval between the posterior margin of the tibial plafond and the dorsal surface of the calcaneal tuberosity (Fig. 10). It is helpful

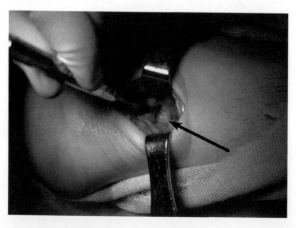

Fig. 10. Posterolateral approach to the ankle for prominent trigonal process of the talus (*arrow*). The osteotome is in the subtalar joint posteriorly.

to palpate and visualize the FHL tendon running medial to the trigonal process of the talus or os trigonum.

The os trigonum is removed by subperiosteal dissection, whereas the lateral tubercle of the posterior process of the talus should be removed with a curved osteotome or rongeur so that the posterior surface of the talus is flush with the posterior surface of the tibia. Excision does not result in lateral subluxation of the FHL tendon because the tendon is contained within a sheath and the line of action of the FHL would cause it to sublux medially if insufficiently constrained.

The posteromedial approach is developed along the tarsal tunnel. The posterior tibialis and flexor digitorum longus tendons should be removed from their sheaths to permit exposure of the deltoid ligament, including the posterior tibiotalar band. The posterior tibial artery and tibial nerve should be retracted posteriorly to approach the FHL, its sheath, and the os trigonum and trigonal process.

The wound is closed in layers, a removable walker boot applied over the dressing, and non–weight bearing enforced for 2 weeks. Range of motion exercises and weight bearing are begun after the incision is adequately healed.

Summary

Ankle instability and ankle impingement are well-known complications of an ankle sprain. Both diagnoses are made primarily by history and physical examination. Ankle instability may resolve with physical therapy, but can require surgical reconstruction. Anatomic reconstruction is preferred whenever possible. Ankle impingement usually requires surgical treatment. Anterior soft tissue impingement and mild bony impingement confined to the tibia can be treated arthroscopically, whereas more severe anterior bony impingement and any form of posterior impingement require an open procedure. Ankle ligament reconstruction and surgical treatment of ankle impingement are reliably effective procedures.

References

[1] Hintermann B. Medial ankle instability. Foot Ankle Clin 2003;8(4):723–38.
[2] Keefe DT, Haddad SL. Subtalar instability. Etiology, diagnosis, and management. Foot Ankle Clin 2002;7(3):577–609.
[3] Martin LP, Wayne JS, Owen JR, et al. Elongation behavior of calcaneofibular and cervical ligaments in a closed kinetic chain: pathomechanics of lateral hindfoot instability. Foot Ankle Int 2002;23(6):515–20.
[4] Sugimoto K, Samoto N, Takakura Y, et al. Varus tilt of the tibial plafond as a factor in chronic ligament instability of the ankle. Foot Ankle Int 1997;18(7):402–5.
[5] Van Bergeyk AB, Younger A, Carson B. CT analysis of hindfoot alignment in chronic lateral ankle instability. Foot Ankle Int 2002;23(1):37–42.
[6] Fortin PT, Guettler J, Manoli A 2nd. Idiopathic cavovarus and lateral ankle instability: recognition and treatment implications relating to ankle arthritis. Foot Ankle Int 2002;23(11):1031–7.

[7] McDermott JE, Scranton PE Jr, Rogers JV. Variations in fibular position, talar length, and anterior talofibular ligament length. Foot Ankle Int 2004;25(9):625–9.

[8] Bassett FH III, Gates HS 3rd, Billys JB, et al. Talar impingement by the anteroinferior tibiofibular ligament. A cause of chronic pain in the ankle after inversion sprain. J Bone Joint Surg Am 1990;72(1):55–9.

[9] Ferkel RD, Karzel RP, Del Pizzo W, et al. Arthroscopic treatment of anterolateral impingement of the ankle. Am J Sports Med 1991;19(5):440–6.

[10] Mosier-La Clair SM, Monroe MT, Manoli A. Medial impingement syndrome of the anterior tibiotalar fascicle of the deltoid ligament on the talus. Foot Ankle Int 2000;21(5):385–91.

[11] Koulouris G, Connell D, Schneider T, et al. Posterior tibiotalar ligament injury resulting in posteromedial impingement. Foot Ankle Int 2003;24(8):575–83.

[12] Paterson RS, Brown JN. The posteromedial impingement lesion of the ankle. A series of six cases. Am J Sports Med 2001;29(5):550–7.

[13] Maquirriain J. Posterior ankle impingement syndrome. J Am Acad Orthop Surg 2005;13(6): 365–71.

[14] Scranton PE Jr, McDermott JE, Rogers JV. The relationship between chronic ankle instability and variations in mortise anatomy and impingement spurs. Foot Ankle Int 2000; 21(8):657–64.

[15] Tol JL, Verheyen CP, van Dijk CN. Arthroscopic treatment of anterior impingement in the ankle. J Bone Joint Surg Br 2001;83(1):9–13.

[16] Molloy S, Solan MC, Bendall SP. Synovial impingement in the ankle. A new physical sign. J Bone Joint Surg Br 2003;85(3):330–3.

[17] Thermann H, Zwipp H, Tscherne H. Treatment algorithm of chronic ankle and subtalar instability. Foot Ankle Int 1997;18(3):163–9.

[18] Beumer A, van Hemert WL, Swierstra BA, et al. A biomechanical evaluation of clinical stress tests for syndesmotic ankle instability. Foot Ankle Int 2003;24(4):358–63.

[19] Tol JL, Verhagen RA, Krips R, et al. The anterior ankle impingement syndrome: diagnostic value of oblique radiographs. Foot Ankle Int 2004;25(2):63–8.

[20] Frost SC, Amendola A. Is stress radiography necessary in the diagnosis of acute or chronic ankle instability? Clin J Sport Med 1999;9(1):40–5.

[21] Lee JW, Suh JS, Huh YM, et al. Soft tissue impingement syndrome of the ankle: diagnostic efficacy of MRI and clinical results after arthroscopic treatment. Foot Ankle Int 2004;25(12): 896–902.

[22] Robinson P, White LM, Salonen D, et al. Anteromedial impingement of the ankle: using MR arthrography to assess the anteromedial recess. AJR Am J Roentgenol 2002;178(3): 601–4.

[23] Robinson P, White LM, Salonen DC, et al. Anterolateral ankle impingement: MR arthrographic assessment of the anterolateral recess. Radiology 2001;221(1):186–90.

[24] Farooki S, Yao L, Seeger LL. Anterolateral impingement of the ankle: effectiveness of MR imaging. Radiology 1998;207(2):357–60.

[25] Rubin DA, Tishkoff NW, Britton CA, et al. Anterolateral soft-tissue impingement in the ankle: diagnosis using MR imaging. AJR Am J Roentgenol 1997;169(3):829–35.

[26] Bureau NJ, Cardinal E, Hobden R, et al. Posterior ankle impingement syndrome: MR imaging findings in seven patients. Radiology 2000;215(2):497–503.

[27] Hamilton WG, Geppert MJ, Thompson FM. Pain in the posterior aspect of the ankle in dancers. Differential diagnosis and operative treatment. J Bone Joint Surg Am 1996;78(10): 1491–500.

[28] Takao M, Oae K, Uchio Y, et al. Anatomical reconstruction of the lateral ligaments of the ankle with a gracilis autograft: a new technique using an interference fit anchoring system. Am J Sports Med 2005;33(6):814–23.

[29] Rosenbaum D, Becker HP, Wilke HJ, et al. Tenodeses destroy the kinematic coupling of the ankle joint complex. A three-dimensional in vitro analysis of joint movement. J Bone Joint Surg Br 1998;80(1):162–8.

[30] Tohyama H, Beynnon BD, Pope MH, et al. Laxity and flexibility of the ankle following reconstruction with the Chrisman-Snook procedure. J Orthop Res 1997;15(5):707–11.

[31] Bahr R, Pena F, Shine J, et al. Biomechanics of ankle ligament reconstruction. An in vitro comparison of the Brostrom repair, Watson-Jones reconstruction, and a new anatomic reconstruction technique. Am J Sports Med 1997;25(4):424–32.

[32] Nimon GA, Dobson PJ, Angel KR, et al. A long-term review of a modified Evans procedure. J Bone Joint Surg Br 2001;83(1):14–8.

[33] Labs K, Perka C, Lang T. Clinical and gait-analytical results of the modified Evans tenodesis in chronic fibulotalar ligament instability. Knee Surg Sports Traumatol Arthrosc 2001;9(2): 116–22.

[34] Krips R, van Dijk CN, Halasi PT, et al. Long-term outcome of anatomical reconstruction versus tenodesis for the treatment of chronic anterolateral instability of the ankle joint: a multicenter study. Foot Ankle Int 2001;22(5):415–21.

[35] Krips R, van Dijk CN, Halasi T, et al. Anatomical reconstruction versus tenodesis for the treatment of chronic anterolateral instability of the ankle joint: a 2- to 10-year follow-up, multicenter study. Knee Surg Sports Traumatol Arthrosc 2000;8(3):173–9.

[36] Hennrikus WL, Mapes RC, Lyons PM, et al. Outcomes of the Chrisman-Snook and modified-Brostrom procedures for chronic lateral ankle instability. A prospective, randomized comparison. Am J Sports Med 1996;24(4):400–4.

[37] Grass R, Rammelt S, Biewener A, et al. Peroneus longus ligamentoplasty for chronic instability of the distal tibiofibular syndesmosis. Foot Ankle Int 2003;24(5):392–7.

[38] Jeys L, Korrosis S, Stewart T, et al. Bone anchors or interference screws? A biomechanical evaluation for autograft ankle stabilization. Am J Sports Med 2004;32(7):1651–9.

[39] Sammarco GJ, Idusuyi OB. Reconstruction of the lateral ankle ligaments using a split peroneus brevis tendon graft. Foot Ankle Int 1999;20(2):97–103.

[40] Urguden M, Soyuncu Y, Ozdemir H, et al. Arthroscopic treatment of anterolateral soft tissue impingement of the ankle: evaluation of factors affecting outcome. Arthroscopy 2005; 21(3):317–22.

[41] Gulish HA, Sullivan RJ, Aronow M. Arthroscopic treatment of soft-tissue impingement lesions of the ankle in adolescents. Foot Ankle Int 2005;26(3):204–7.

[42] Kim SH, Ha KI. Arthroscopic treatment for impingement of the anterolateral soft tissues of the ankle. J Bone Joint Surg Br 2000;82(7):1019–21.

[43] Akseki D, Pinar H, Bozkurt M, et al. The distal fascicle of the anterior inferior tibio-fibular ligament as a cause of anterolateral ankle impingement: results of arthroscopic resection. Acta Orthop Scand 1999;70(5):478–82.

[44] DeBerardino TM, Arciero RA, Taylor DC. Arthroscopic treatment of soft-tissue impingement of the ankle in athletes. Arthroscopy 1997;13(4):492–8.

[45] Tol JL, van Dijk CN. Etiology of the anterior ankle impingement syndrome: a descriptive anatomical study. Foot Ankle Int 2004;25(6):382–6.

[46] van Dijk CN, Tol JL, Verheyen CC. A prospective study of prognostic factors concerning the outcome of arthroscopic surgery for anterior ankle impingement. Am J Sports Med 1997; 25(6):737–45.

[47] Coull R, Raffiq T, James LE, et al. Open treatment of anterior impingement of the ankle. J Bone Joint Surg Br 2003;85(4):550–3.

[48] Berberian WS, Hecht PJ, Wapner KL, et al. Morphology of tibiotalar osteophytes in anterior ankle impingement. Foot Ankle Int 2001;22(4):313–7.

[49] Henderson I, La Valette D. Ankle impingement: combined anterior and posterior impingement syndrome of the ankle. Foot Ankle Int 2004;25(9):632–8.

ELSEVIER
SAUNDERS

Foot Ankle Clin N Am
12 (2007) 197–213

FOOT AND
ANKLE CLINICS

Index

Note: Page numbers of article titles are in **boldface** type.

A

Achilles tendon, contracture of, ankle salvage osteotomy and, 10–11
in PTTD staging, 17

Achilles tendonitis, with calcaneal fractures, 2

Agility total ankle cutting guide, in osteochondral allograft reconstruction, of talar dome, 48

American Orthopaedic Foot and Ankle Society (AOFAS) score, post-ankle salvage osteotomy, 5
post-calcaneal malunion correction, 130–131, 133–134
post-calcaneal osteotomy, for varus ankle, 160
post-distraction arthroplasty, for ankle arthritis, 29–30
post-osteochondral allograft reconstruction, for ankle articular segment deficits, 52
post-talus neck malunion correction, 146–147

Amputations, for combined subtalar and ankle arthritis, 71

Anatomic reduction, of talus neck fractures, 138–139, 141
open. See *Open reduction and internal fixation (ORIF)*.

Angle of Gissane, in calcaneus, 126
fractures and, 127, 129

Ankle arthritis, biomechanics of, 30–31
arthroplasty and, 31–32
distraction arthroplasty for, **29–39**.
See also *Distraction arthroplasty*.
in valgus ankle, 19–20
post-talus neck fracture, reconstruction for, **137–151**.
See also *Talus neck fracture*.
salvage osteotomy for, **1–13**
fibular, 5–8
hindfoot, 8–11

midfoot, 8–11
summary of, 12
supramalleolar, 1–5
subtalar arthritis combined with, **57–73**
as difficult to treat, 57, 64, 71
biomechanics of, 58
causes of, 57–58
nonoperative treatment of, 58–59
operative treatment of, 59–71
amputation in, 71
arthroplasty in, 68–69
salvage of failed, 70–71
complications with, 69–70
goal of, 60
indications for, 59–60
tibiotalocalcaneal arthrodesis in, gait and, 68
key concepts of, 60
postoperative management of, 65
results of, 65–68
techniques for, 60–65
surgical options for, 29–30, 38

Ankle (tibiotalar) arthrodesis, 77
for varus ankle, surgical technique for, 168–170
total ankle replacement versus, 165–168, 173–174
nonunion of, 78
clinical studies of, 80–82

Ankle articular injuries, arthrodesis for, 41, 45, 48
calcaneal fractures as, 126–127
osteochondral allograft reconstruction of, **41–55**. See also *Ankle articular segment deficits*.
patterns of, 43
talus neck fracture as. See also *Talus neck fracture*.
reconstruction for, **137–151**
total ankle arthroplasty for, 41, 48

Moving?

Make sure your subscription moves with you!

To notify us of your new address, find your **Clinics Account Number** (located on your mailing label above your name), and contact customer service at:

E-mail: elspcs@elsevier.com

800-654-2452 (subscribers in the U.S. & Canada)
407-345-4000 (subscribers outside of the U.S. & Canada)

Fax number: 407-363-9661

Elsevier Periodicals Customer Service
6277 Sea Harbor Drive
Orlando, FL 32887-4800

*To ensure uninterrupted delivery of your subscription, please notify us at least 4 weeks in advance of move.